OSTEOPATHY

RESEARCH AND PRACTICE

A. T. STILL

Published by Left of Brain Books

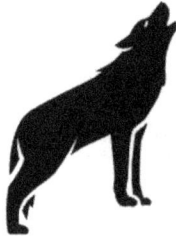

Copyright © 2021 Left of Brain Books

ISBN 978-1-396-32150-4

First Edition

Table of Contents

THIS book is respectfully dedicated to the *Grand Architect and Builder of the Universe*; to *Osteopaths* and all other persons who believe that the *First Great Master Mechanic* left nothing unfinished in the machinery of His masterpiece—*Man*—that is necessary for his comfort or longevity.

PREFACE

In working out the general scheme of this book I have considered the human body in sections, or regions. I have classified the effects of abnormalities of the human body, or the so-called diseases, upon a basis of nerve and blood supply and the region affected. Often the line of separation cannot be closely drawn, as will be seen in my discussion of the condition. I have considered the most general diseased conditions of the regions of the head, neck, thorax, abdomen and pelvis. Some conditions being more extensive in their effects do not properly fall into any of these classes but belong to the region above the diaphragm. Others belong to the region below the diaphragm; while others general in character, are spoken of as spinal. For convenience in referring to contagious diseases and fevers I have grouped them under a separate heading.

I have omitted all cuts and pictures because the reader of my practice is supposed to have in his mind an image of every bone, muscle, nerve, organ and part of the human body. His thorough anatomical and physiological acquaintance with the body makes it useless to have illustrations in this work. On your table are fully illustrated works on anatomy by able authors. Keep well posted on anatomy because the osteopath reasons from his mechanical knowledge of anatomy.

I have quoted many definitions from Dunglison's and Dorland's latest works. We consider them standard authorities and herewith give them credit and thanks.

I have given you from my many years of experience and observation what I consider some of the underlying causes of these so-called diseases, which are seen as effects in the different regions of the body, together with my method of treating such causes.

While I do not propose to follow in the old medical tracks, I want here and now to give my love and pay my respects to those doctors who are now in their graves, as well as to those living, who have tried honestly to bring relief to suffering humanity. I agree with what has been and is now the opinion of many of them, that the world would be just as well off or even better off (with very slight exception) had there never been a system of drug medication.

I was born and raised to respect and confide in the remedial power of drugs, but after many years of practice in close conformity to the dictations of the very best medical authors and in consultation with representatives of the various schools, I failed to get from drugs the results hoped for and I was face to face with the evidence that medication was not only untrustworthy but was dangerous.

The mechanical principles on which osteopathy is based are as old as the universe. I discovered them while I was in Kansas. You can call this discovery accidental or purely philosophical. I was in the practice of medicine and had been for several years. I treated my patients as other doctors did. A part of them got well and a part died. Others both old and young got sick and got well without the assistance of the medical doctor.

As I was an educated engineer of five years' schooling I began to look at the human framework as a machine and examine all its parts to see if I could find any variation from the truly normal among its journals, belts, pulleys and escape pipes. I began to experiment with man's body as a master mechanic would when he had in his charge any machinery which needed to be kept perfectly adjusted and in line in order to get perfect work. There are many ways by which a machine may be adjusted. An osteopathic operator is not expected to depend on any one method or manipulation for the adjustment of a bone.

I worked along faithfully, patiently and hopefully, finding out that the human body was just as liable to strains and variations as a steam engine, and that after correcting the strains and variations health was sure to follow. I was many years philosophizing, comparing and noticing results which followed taking off strains and pressures. I was surprised to see that fever, congestion and all irregularities gave way, health returned, and the results were good and satisfactory.

I found mechanical causes for disordered functioning, or poor work of the head, neck, thorax, abdomen, pelvis or extremities. I adjusted the bony framework and secured such good results that I was encouraged to keep on and on until now I can truthfully say that I am satisfied that osteopathy is the natural way by which all of the diseases to which the human family is heir can be relieved, and a large majority of them cured.

Osteopathy is based on the perfection of Nature's work. When all parts of the human body are in-line we have health. When they are not the effect is disease. When the parts are readjusted disease gives place to health. The work of the osteopath is to adjust the body from the abnormal to the normal; then the abnormal condition gives place to the normal and health is the result of the normal condition.

The God of Nature is the fountain of skill and wisdom and the mechanical work done in all natural bodies is the result of absolute knowledge. Man cannot add anything to this perfect work nor improve the functioning of the normal body. Disease is an effect only, and a positive proof that a belt is off, a journal bent, or a cog broken or caught. Man's power to cure is good as far as he has a knowledge of the right or normal position, and so far as he has the skill to adjust the bones, muscles and ligaments and give freedom to nerves, blood, secretions and excretions, and no farther. We credit God with wisdom and skill to perform perfect work on the house of life in which man lives. It is only justice that God should receive this credit and we are ready to adjust the parts and trust the results.

I want to thank my three brothers, my wife and my children for their aid and encouragement in this work. I want also to thank all persons who have given me a kind word, a smile of encouragement, a handshake, or bade me Godspeed during the period of time in which I was prosecuting the unfolding of this science which I believe to be the living truth and which has demonstrated itself as such.

In conclusion I want to say that I extend my love to all persons who by word or act have encouraged the unfolding of the science of osteopathy; also to those who will in time to come receive benefit from the science and send back a thought of gratitude to the pioneer who has tried to blaze the way. I thank you one and all from the inner depths of my soul and I wish each of you Godspeed.

A. T. STILL.

INTRODUCTION

When reading this treatise on diseases, their cause and cure from an osteopathic standpoint, I think the reader will soon observe that I am talking to him. I want him to listen and think. I do not expect to quote Shakespeare, Robert Burns, nor any other author save Nature. I speak from practical experience in Nature's school and from the philosophy of an American who is neither ashamed nor afraid to say or do what he thinks truthful honesty demands.

This work is strictly American. The development and unfolding of the many and great conveniences known to exist in this country are due to and the result of the skill of the American mechanic. Any person wishing to know this is the truth has only to acquaint himself with the reports of the patent office of the United States, which, if I am rightly informed, has issued many more patents to its inventors than any other country or government.

It was the inventive mind that first thought out and put into execution the application of steam and electricity for all useful purposes both on land and sea. The inventor's head is high above all other heads because his work shows that he thought and studied on cause and effect. He reasons, works and waits the demonstration of facts to prove the truth of his reasoning. To the inventive thinker we owe our ease and safety when on sea and land; to the inventor we are indebted for fuller cribs, fatter hogs, sheep and cattle, because many of his inventions are in the interest of the farmer, the horticulturist, and so on throughout the list.

Without asking any reader's pardon I use the English language because it is plain, and I hate the cobwebs of delusive words which have gotten into all of our medical books on surgery, midwifery and general practice. The most abominable nuisance I find between man and his receipt of knowledge is that great cobweb of delusive and incomprehensible words that some doctors feel called upon to use when they try to talk to an American thinker about such important subjects as diseases of the human body. He talks at great length and says nothing to the point. The listener becomes disgusted because the doctor fails to demonstrate his claims, in his practice. His theory is a failure as proven by the results.

I want it understood that I look upon the treating of effects as being as unwarranted as it would be for the firemen of a city to fight the smoke and pay no attention to the cause that produced it. Is such teaching wise? You may answer the question. I think it is a great mistake to ignore man as a machine—the latest, best, and the one pronounced not only good but "very good"—a product of the greatest architectural mechanic of the universe, God.

This book has been written under a physical protest, my health not being good enough for me to enjoy the place of an author on any subject, but osteopathy is a science which I think can be explained only on a mechanical basis. I know this book is far from perfection, and it is my hope and wish that every osteopath will go on and on in search for scientific facts as they relate to the human mechanism and health, and to an ever-extended unfolding of Nature's truths and laws.

I have no doubt of the willingness of others to write in my place and take this labor off my shoulders, but that knowledge which I have obtained for and against the principles and practice of osteopathy during the past fifty years cannot be furnished by any one who has not had the experiences in the work and a life-long observation. Thus I write.

It is my object to tell what I know to be the truth without using the words "possibly," "however," "may be so," or any other evasive phrases, such as are usually applied to undemonstrable theories. In their place I give you what I think are facts to which I can say "yes," "no," "I did," "you can," and so on.

With this short introduction I leave you to study and practice the philosophy of osteopathy as here set forth, governing yourselves accordingly and forming conclusions of your own, based upon the day-by-day's unfolding of the science.

OSTEOPATHIC FUNDAMENTALS

WHY I AM AN OSTEOPATH.

The Medical Incubator has had an unbroken privilege in choice of places, the very best oil, the best thermometers, the best attention and also the prayers of the whole world for all ages. The box has been kept filled with eggs during all this time hoping that a chicken could be hatched to take the name that had long been waiting for him, the Medical Game Cock, whose spurs and force could successfully combat the Cock of Disease. The chicken hoped for has never been hatched. This incubator has had eggs put in it from all the hens that have laid nostrums and they have failed to hatch a single specific rooster for any disease. It is estimated that five hundred new eggs or nostrums are put under this hen or incubator every month, only to fail—they hatch, rot, burst and stink.

We have had pathologists, chemists, allopaths, homeopaths, electropaths, waterpaths until it would make you tired to listen to the 'paths, and all have proven to be lamentable failures. We have listened to their request and advice for thousands of years and the promises they have made have been abortions. From them we have nothing to hope. Our road is straight through the woods. Old trees must fall, stumps must be taken out, trees of life and hope must be planted to declare the intelligence of the Architect of Life. The osteopaths are the army all ready to combat. Our captain is the God of Nature who has never failed in any of His plans or specifications, and His promise is be thou faithful unto the end and the reward shall be good health every day, and He says, hope thou and Me.

Allow me to say that I love the old doctors for their faithfulness; I pity them for their universal failure. I know their intentions were good. If any one of the 'pathies or the whole of them, had produced a single panacea for any disease it would be different, but I have spent a life in acquainting myself with what they say and do, and I think I would be dishonest to the youth, the middle-aged and to the coming generations to recommend that which I know is not true. I want to emphasize that my vote is now, first, last and all the time, and has been for the last thirty-five years, against the use of anything but Nature's remedies for treating the sick.

The special panacea, surgery, which has been a growing curse for many years is the desire for the unwarranted use of the knife, the excuse for which is the effort to seek a cure for this and that disease by mutilating the body and throwing away that which is useful and should be retained as a part of the human body for its longevity and comfort. The medical doctor reasons that the body has chemicals in it that have to be met with other chemicals or poisons. The drugs which are chemical products have been administered according to his direction and have failed to relieve a suffering head, neck, chest, abdomen, pelvis, or any organ.

The symptomatologist comes forward and describes, classifies and names the disease and prescribes his remedies. We ask him why he did not give us those names a week sooner. His answer is "we have to wait long enough for the disease to develop before we are warranted in giving names." This is a fairly good acknowledgment that he did not know what the disease was. Does the doctor say he did not dope with the same blindness? No, he says "I dosed and dosed freely for a number of days until I found I had smallpox to contend with. Had I known it was smallpox in the beginning my treatment would have been different." The osteopath has his own symptomatology. He seeks the cause, removes the obstruction and lets Nature's remedy—arterial blood—be the doctor; and when his patient is cured, he has in his system no blindly administered medicine with which he must contend. He who treats symptoms is the man who fights disease with specifics, and if intelligent and honest he will say "No specific has ever been found for any disease." This is the claim of the sages of all schools, and I ask myself the question, why should I follow such practice?

WHY I WRITE THIS BOOK.

I have but one object in writing on this subject, which is to present the truth as nearly as, possible and assist and aid the osteopath to reason from the effect he sees to the cause which, in many cases, is unseen. He should never dally with effects but ever go back to the cause which when corrected results in a disappearance of the effect. It is my hope that the osteopath may be hereby better prepared to do his work.

Osteopathy is a science. Its use is in the healing of the afflicted. It is a philosophy which embraces surgery, obstetrics and general practice. An osteopath must be a man of reason and prove his talk by his work. He has no use for theories unless they are demonstrated. Osteopathy is to me a very sacred science. It is sacred because it is a healing power through all nature. I am very jealous of it and will accept nothing from any man's pen as a truthful presentation of this science unless he courts investigation and proves by demonstration that every statement is a truth. It is a science that asks no favors or friendship of the old schools; they have long since acknowledged they have never discovered a single trustworthy remedy for any disease. Having been familiar myself for years with all their methods and having experimented with them I became disheartened and disgusted and dropped them.

Many fairly good writers on other subjects have made very unsatisfactory presentations of this philosophy. I think a writer on osteopathy should speak from his own experience and keep his scissors out of the text books of the old schools which stand condemned as fallacious and untrustworthy in time of need. It is wrong for any author to write a book which he claims to be a work on osteopathy but which is simply the sayings of those who do not know anything of it.

I am proud of osteopathic surgery which never uses a knife for the removal of tumors of the breast, abdomen or any other part of the body, until the arterial supply and venous drainage have failed to restore vitality and reduce the system and organs to their normal functioning. Through the arterial supply and the venous drain age a large per cent of tumors of the abdomen and breast will vanish in the hands of a trustworthy and philosophical osteopathic doctor. Osteopaths should never dread to meet the climatic or the diseases of the four seasons of the year. He should go into the combat with his knowledge of physiology and anatomy and conduct his patients safely through fevers of all types. He should never fear to take a case of diphtheria, scarlet fever, tonsillitis, sore throat, measles, pneumonia, typhoid fever, erysipelas, etc., if he is called in reasonable time. With the knowledge of the function of the arterial blood to build and the venous blood to carry off, he should hold himself at all times to the tenets of osteopathy, and allow no accumulation of fluids to be retained in any gland of the face, neck or other portion of the body. He should combat these conditions and relieve and cure his patient without the assistance of any adjuncts more than cleanliness.

About adjuncts I want to say that when an osteopath explores the human body for the cause of disease he knows he is dealing with complicated perfection. He must master anatomy and physiology and have a fairly good knowledge of chemistry; then he can reason from the effect to the cause that gives rise to the abnormal condition or disease. He cures by the correction of all hindering causes to the normal flow of blood and other fluids. An osteopath reasons from his knowledge of anatomy. He compares the work of the abnormal body with the work of the normal body. Adjuncts are not necessary to the osteopath. An osteopath who depends on the use of wet sheets, cold or hot, forgets that the arteries, veins and nerves are responsible for normal temperature and repairs. If he is an up-to-date osteopath his hand is his thermometer; his hand is his syringe. An osteopath kills diphtheria worms with the club of reason dipped in pure arterial blood.

I want to impress upon the reader of this book that I will give no undemonstrable theory. I will give in detail a full description of how to proceed from start to finish in handling the diseases of the head, neck, chest, abdomen, pelvis and limbs, and just how I have opened and prosecuted the treatment for many diseases to a successful termination. All of the bacteriology that I want or need is a good knowledge of man's anatomy, of the functioning of his organs and how to know the cause of the friction that has produced the disease; then I relieve it.

As this science is very new to a great many at the present date, it is my desire to give such instructions as can be used and demonstrated. This is an effort at the beginning to write reliable and instructive osteopathic literature. I feel that the time has come and a demand with it that a book of instruction be written which will be a guide by which the student can proceed as a thinker, operator and successful osteopathic doctor. For this reason I have written as far as possible in the plainest language. Furthermore, I have used simple, plain language so that those of the laity who desire to read my book will understand it.

OUR PLATFORM.

It should be known where osteopathy stands and what it stands for. A political party has a platform that all may know its position in regard to matters of public importance, what it stands for and what principles it advocates. The osteopath should make his position just as clear to the public. He should let the public know, in his platform, what he advocates in his campaign against disease. Our position can be tersely stated in the following planks:

First: We believe in sanitation and hygiene.

Second: We are opposed to the use of drugs as remedial agencies.

Third: We are opposed to vaccination.

Fourth: We are opposed to the use of serums in the treatment of disease. Nature furnishes its own serum if we know how to deliver them.

Fifth: We realize that many cases require surgical treatment and therefore advocate it as a last resort. We believe many surgical operations are unnecessarily performed and that many operations can be avoided by osteopathic treatment.

Sixth: The osteopath does not depend on electricity, X—radiance, hydrotherapy or other adjuncts, but relies on osteopathic measures in the treatment of disease.

Seventh: We have a friendly feeling for other non-drug, natural methods of healing, but we do not in corporate any other methods into our system. We are all opposed to drugs; in that respect at least, all natural, unharmful methods occupy the same ground. The fundamental principles of osteopathy are different from those of any other system and the cause of disease is considered from one standpoint, viz.: disease is the result of anatomical abnormalities followed by physiological discord. To cure disease the abnormal parts must be adjusted to the normal; therefore other methods that are entirely different in principle have no place in the osteopathic system.

Eighth: Osteopathy is an independent system and can be applied to all conditions of disease, including purely surgical cases, and in these cases surgery is but a branch of osteopathy.

Ninth: We believe that our therapeutic house is just large enough for osteopathy and that when other methods are brought in just that much osteopathy must move out.

THE BROTHERHOOD OF LIFE.

Let us reason that at conception every organ of the whole human body enters one great labor union. They labor and do faithful and good work until one member of the union is mistreated. Then the whole brotherhood comes to a halt to consult, and it never compromises, until the doctor sets all things right, or apologizes for his failure and calls counsel. The head, neck, chest, abdomen, limbs and all organs belong to the brotherhood of labor, and they are commissioned to show perfect work and good health. They do this when everything is in order and there is plenty of nourishment and a reasonable amount of rest and amusement.

The operator who explores for the true cause of so many deadly effects on the system should keep in mind that any organ when injured by atmospheric changes, wounds, bruises, mental shocks, etc., very often produces such changes as result in death. Local shocks affect the whole system, the nerve and blood supply to every part of the body. They disable or confuse the secretory and excretory systems and the fluids retained become deadly poisons. In many cases a nail driven through the foot will produce lockjaw as an effect of that shock, and death is the result. Extremes of atmospheric temperatures so shock the pleurae, lungs, pulmonary nerves and blood-vessels as to produce stagnation of fluids and result in tuberculosis and death. Or the shock shows its effect on the brain, heart, stomach, bowels, kidneys, liver, spleen or any other organ and then we have a strike on until the nerves of the injured organ or part are free from all oppression and have a chance to repair the damage.

A jar or slip of the hip produces an inflammation the result of which will extend over the whole body. There is stagnation and fermentation of the fluids and a cheesy deposit is the result. Thus we see a cause of tuberculosis, local and general. The blood in the hip becomes poisonous and is carried to all parts of the body, and there is general weakness. In this way tuberculosis of the lungs can result. The importance of injuries to the hip are too much overlooked. To the osteopath it should be a subject of the deepest thought.

It matters not to a mechanic whether you analyze the blood. He hunts for the cause of friction and when he finds it he removes that cause. If there are bony variations, if muscles or nerves are oppressed, he removes the cause and

14

the result is harmony and it is felt throughout the system. Because of his thorough acquaintance with the structure and functioning of the whole system, the mechanic can tell you the cause of tuberculosis, kidney diseases, etc. The answer of a mechanic is "yes," or "no," without a "however" or "maybe-so" and he proves his knowledge by demonstration.

No author, except the mechanic, has been able to give the cause, effect and cure of such diseases. A mechanic will not send an asthmatic to the mountains. He knows the cause, adjusts the bones and the asthma disappears. In lung trouble if the patient comes before general decomposition of the lungs has occurred and while the recuperative powers of the body are in full possession, the result is the same. I think the most important advice I can give the student of osteopathy and the operator who objects to old theories and uses his head as his day star of reason is, to look upon the human body as an organized brotherhood of laborers. The business of the operator is to keep peace and harmony throughout the whole brotherhood. He is a worthy osteopath who realizes the great importance of this truth, and practices it.

AN OBJECT IN NATURE'S WORK.

Nature's object in fetal life is the production of a machine which when completed is sent forth for a purpose. In this shop the highest order of architecture and construction of substance and form is completed, and sent forth from the first conception to the atmospheric world which we will call the second conception. The hour of birth is the beginning of intellectual conception when a new being, the intellectual man, begins to develop. When first born the product of conception is an intellectual blank, but has the power to conceive and obey all of the laws of knowledge of the physical world.

He grows in knowledge from the hour of his birth to the day of his death. His knowledge is received by the five senses. He sees something which is his first item of knowledge. He hears something, and as he grows older he feels, tastes and smells. Through these five senses the seeds of knowledge and reason are developed.

He was attached to the placenta and stayed there until the highest order of physical perfection was completed. He left the placenta behind as dead matter. He left it as a part of the machinery that produced the physical form of the intellectual man. He has severed the connections with the producing shop for all time.

I will now, ask what is his second condition? Is not this physical form, this intellectual man, a placenta in principle? A placenta for the purpose of constructing a greater being which we will call life? What is death but a birth from the second placenta to which life has been attached? If this philosophy is true, death is only the delivery of the finished life whose perfection is far superior to the intellectual man, the maternal house of construction, which is left behind. It is a known fact that human life is progressive and that it prepares to proceed with the labor of accumulation and practice of knowledge. It is reasonable to conclude that after what is known as physical death, the life is then and there qualified to enter the higher school to continue its mental development. In all this Nature had some great object in view. My conclusion is that immortality is the design or object of Nature's God in the production of man.

Notwithstanding that all nature is a well-prepared engine, that the plan and specification for ruling and governing the whole universe is and has been right before us, that men, fishes, beasts and all vegetables are constant exhibitions of some kind of engine for some purpose, yet, man's mental eyes do not open to behold the perfection of the Architect and Builder. His eyes do not open to see that man when completed is a perfect machine, constructed for a purpose, and that nourishment and rest are the requirements for its work of construction and motion, both of body and mind.

As a mechanical engineer who has lived a long time in both worlds, the world of medication and guess work and the world of a mechanic who has long occupied the seat of an engineer and conducted the repairing and running of the locomotive of human life, I want to say, that I left medication as a healing art because by long experience I proved to my own satisfaction that the medical man has no claim to be called scientific. When I proclaimed that man is the proof of the work that shows a perfect plan, a perfect specification, a perfect construction with all parts and principles to demonstrate that the human body is a machine of unlimited perfection in performing the duties for which it was constructed, whether physical or intellectual, the world said "No," and "Pshaw."

For thirty-five years I have observed man's body with the eyes of a mechanic so that I could behold and see the execution of the work for which it was designed, and I have come to this conclusion: The better I am acquainted with the parts and principles of this machine—man—the louder it speaks that from start to finish it is the work of some trustworthy architect; and all the mysteries concerning health disappear just in proportion to man's acquaintance with this sacred product, its parts and principles, separate, united or in action. It is an honor to its Builder who should be respected for the perfection set forth and shown by man as a product of Life and its constructive intelligence. I consider man the answer to the question, does Nature prove its perfection by its work? I say yes, and treat the human body as a machine should be treated by a mechanic. I have found that there is no equivocation, no "may-be-so's"; the answer is absolute. The product says, "I am the answer to all questions that can possibly be asked by the anatomical, the physiological and the chemical conductor of this engine, whether it is in the normal or the abnormal condition."

SYSTEMS AND SUCCESSES.

Nature moves by system in all her works. She succeeds in all because her plans are perfect. Her designs have an object as their day star, and with her eyes fixed on the plan the effect is seen to follow. The body of man or beast is made for a purpose and to get results. The nature-system must show in all parts of the body. The system of producing blood must be so perfect that all parts can run without obstruction. Food taken into the stomach is passed through each process by a perfect system and order. Force or power to move and run the parts must be provided for. Nerves of every kind are a part of the system of force and action.

Then again we see system in the size and place of every structure and the manner in which each is connected to the heart and the brain by perfect ganglionized systems. Every blood-vessel is accompanied and controlled by forces suited to the system of blood supply. We must have good action or meet bad results. The heart does the hard work of delivering blood to all parts of the body and must also be fed; hence the demand for the coronary arterial system and the perfect order of its blood and nerve supply without which the heart will fail in its functioning in the whole system of blood supply because it has not been kept normal in size. In order to inspect the heart for cause of any failure to do perfect work the osteopath must know the form, place, function and action of each organ. He must keep all parts in perfect position before he can expect the heart to report "all is well." He must keep all channels open for blood and other fluids to pass and return because no variation can be allowed without confusion and bad effects resulting.

The osteopath who succeeds best does so because he looks to Nature for knowledge and obeys her teaching, then he gets good results. He is often amazed to see how faithfully Nature sticks to system. A few years spent in the school of Nature teaches the osteopath that principles govern the universe, and he must obey all orders, or fail to cure his patients. We say disease when we should say effect; for disease is the effect of a change in the parts of the physical body. Disease in an abnormal body is just as natural as is health when all parts are in place. One asks how we may know the normal. Surely we know when the hat fits the head and the pants the legs. We should know the normal places of all bones, and their uses; how one is attached to another; where blood and nerve supply come from and how. If we do not, we must learn or we will blunder and fail, because no variation will be allowed if we get health.

If the laws of the universe are systematic according to kind, then we must observe and follow each system faithfully if we expect to change effects, because every change in cause gives a new effect. The universe is governed by that law. That law is life. Its attributes we see or know by their effects as shown in worlds and beings, and ailments both mental and physical. If the lungs pass final sentence on the blood's perfection then we must keep them wholly normal. We know the heart delivers without regard to quality of blood.

NATURE AS AN ARCHITECT.

Definition.—(1). An architect is one skilled in practical architecture; one whose profession it is to devise the plans and ornamentation of buildings or other structures and direct their construction. (2). One who contrives, plans, makes, or builds up something.

—*Standard Dictionary.*

Is God an architect? If so why not be governed by the plan, specification, building and engineering of that Architect in our work as healers? When we conform to and work by the laws and specifications of this Architect, we get the results required. This is the foundation stone on which osteopathy stands and has stood for thirty-five years.

I want to impress on the mind of the operator that when he is competent and works after Nature's plan and specification he can so repair the human engine that it will do all of the work necessary to animal life. When you have no surgical wounds or injuries the result will be just what you expect, no more, no less. When you have adjusted the human body to the degree of absolute perfection, all parts in place, none excepted, then perfect health is your answer. Nature has no apology to offer. It does the work if you know how to line up the parts; then food and rest are all that is required.

I have not only worked to relieve and cure the sick, but I have had both eyes open all the time to find a defect in Nature's work, its object, its plan, its specification, its building and its engineering; so far I have failed to find a variation from perfection.

MAN'S BODY IS LIKE UNTO A CITY.

Let us say that each person is a well organized city and reason by comparison that the city makes all the workshops necessary to produce such machinery as is required for the health and comfort of its inhabitants. Each organ is a laborer of skill and belongs to the union of Perfect Work. Each laborer or organ must be in perfect health, or some degree of failure, a beginning of universal shortage in perfect work throughout the system or city, will be the result.

When the city is in bad condition and we have imperfect work on the part of the mechanics of the sewage department, it will grow worse and worse daily. When the excretory system is not kept clean the city becomes filthy and unhealthy. Thus the various kinds of diseases or plagues begin from a cause and destroy the whole city.

Just as a filthy sewer will produce disease in the whole city, so the failure of one organ will produce disease of the whole body, and the salvation of the city or body, depends on your mechanical philosophy and work. What osteopath is so intellectually blind as not to see the truth of this statement? Osteopathy has no place for the masseur, but for the mechanic of first water, endowed by nature and well qualified by practice. The osteopath's word is not to be accepted until he demonstrates what he has asserted.

ORGANS AS FUNCTIONARIES.

Success in any work will show the foundation on which the successful man or woman stood and without which no one can hope to succeed. When we treat diseases of the whole system we must have a foundation or fail. The osteopath's foundation is, that all the blood must move all the time in all parts to and from all organs. The organs must have good blood all the time and plenty of it. The blood must do its work and return to the heart and lungs and there leave its impurities, then return as pure blood to do its work again and so continue through life.

The foundation on which the osteopath stands should show a reason why disease is simply an effect. Until the explorer hunts for and finds the cause or friction that has produced the effect, his labors will be hard and unsatisfactory. In order to help in the search for cause we will now present to you some of the organs as functionaries. No two organs are alike, therefore their responsibilities are different.

The human body as a whole is a functionary with duties to perform. The brain is a functionary whose duty is to prepare and send forth through the nervous system the forces and fluids necessary to the action of organs of the whole system, none excepted, and that function must be performed to the degree of healthy perfection. The brain secretes, prepares and excretes; and if the brain receives an injury from surgical or other cause, it is not reasonable to suppose that that brain can make the pure and wholesome fluid for the nervous system which is necessary in order to have a healthy and undisturbed condition of the body. We must be sure that every bone is lined up and in its proper position, not held to the right nor the left by any muscular contraction which would follow irritation to the muscle or its nerves. The nervous system comes in as an individualized functionary whose duty it is to receive and distribute nervous forces to the whole system. The heart is another functionary whose function it is to receive the blood and distribute it through the arterial system to nourish and build every organ and every atom of flesh in the whole body. All parts must have blood and all are dependent for their nourishment upon the arterial.

Then another functionary arises and says, "I am the venous system. My commission and order is to return the exhausted blood back to the heart and unite the chyle and other substances mixed and thrown to the lungs for purification and separation, and carry it up to the degree of living arterial blood." The lung is one of the highest functionaries of the whole system. According to every method of reasoning the lung comes in as the GREAT I AM of living blood. As a functionary its duty is to prepare and return to the heart the pure substances known as arterial blood. The lungs secrete and excrete. Should this functionary fail to receive the proper force from the nervous system it is to be expected that the arterial blood will be of an impure and inferior quality. Thus all organs will show disease in proportion to the quality of arterial blood upon which they are fed and from which they receive their nourishment. In order to have good arterial blood the lungs must receive good wholesome food from the abdomen. If they do not, a failure in proportion to the impurities of the chyle, and so on, will be seen.

Would it be reasonable to expect to keep in a healthy condition with impure blood as nourishment? Would you expect the arterial blood to build and keep up a healthy kidney with poor food substance? This same law of reasoning applies to the spleen, pancreas, stomach, omentum, peritoneum, bowels, bladder, uterus, and all parts or organs of the abdominal viscera. Thus you will reason that typhoid fever is not a disease of the bowels but a failure of the lungs to send forth pure arterial blood to repair and keep the bowels in normal condition, the effect of which is disease. This is my conclusion. Would you expect the uterus or bladder, the bowels great or small, the pancreas, the spleen or peritoneum to execute their work as functionaries without the necessary nourishment to enable them to perform the duties incumbent upon them? As a mechanic I answer no. As a philosopher who is able to reason you will also say no; and you will see that the garden, the fountain of life, is the lung, and that every atom of arterial blood is sent forth as ripe seed grown in the garden of life, the lungs.

Let us go a little higher. The lung itself has to be fed. The heart, the brain, the whole nervous system all must have perfectly pure nourishment or fail to perform their function just in proportion to the degree of imperfection found in the blood. The eye, the tongue, the ear and the respiratory system each is a responsible functionary and must execute its work to the degree of perfection, and I ask you how it can do this and live on impure substances? The lung has done the best it could and has made the blood as high in quality as was possible for it to do because the nervous system has refused to act in the abdomen and the abdomen has failed to send forth a high grade of chyle.

BLOOD SEED.

Truth has no cause to fear opinions. It wants no flattery. It neither loves nor hates. It is food and comfort. The osteopath is the blacksmith at his anvil. The blacksmith proves his wit by his work. An osteopath shows his skill by the result of his work. A hen shows results by the worms she scratches out. Talk is talk, but the biscuits speak for the cook. A horse may not have a beautiful body, but if he has the "git there" in his heels, he is the horse that wins the prize. If you want to show your wife's brains, bring in her babes. They will be the "show up" for all the talk. If "dad" is not a fool they will be bright as the new moon.

Every atom of blood when sent forth from the lungs is a living seed, as much so as the seed of any shrub, flower or tree in all nature. When those atoms are delivered to the proper soil in the human body they grow and that which is added or is a product of its growth is as real as the substance that we see or find in the cabbage or the lettuce or in any vegetable whatsoever. When these seeds or atoms are not normal, they are not appropriated in the human system, but are refused or thrown off by the body tissues and become the active agents in the production of disease. Because of the quality of life imparted to them whilst in the lungs they will grow even in a lower stratum; and when they do not find healthful soil or conditions they will grow in diseased soil.

That the atoms of blood can and do grow and multiply in size and do vital work is no longer doubted; and the surgeon who grafts skin or flesh in cases of burns or injuries knows that if the adjacent parts are normal he will have vital union because of the seed property of the blood atoms. With this quality the atoms acting as seeds multiply when in soil to suit their growth. The success of skin grafting depends on good blood and sound flesh. The surgeon well knows that when the arterial atoms or seeds fall in diseased fluids bad union, is the result, for the atoms become diseased and his work is a failure. Then if he takes of such local blood and places it under growing conditions to suit, he sees living atoms move. Thus you have your microorganisms. They are the developed atoms of life or the seed generated in the lungs and returned to the heart and sent forth as arterial blood which is nothing more nor less than the seed of life. Thus the philosopher sees no mystery in the so-called micro-organisms of disease.

In discussing diseases of the lungs, heart, bowels or other organs we must decide one very important question. Where do the atoms of blood receive that degree of perfection which is the seedlike property of the atom by which when planted in proper soil it will vegetate, grow and produce what we call tissue, bone, muscle and all constructed substances? Now the most important of all known questions presents itself to the philosopher. Where is the garden spot that gives the seedlike property to the atoms of blood, if it is not the lungs? According to my method of reasoning the responsibility of the lung is as great as that of any other organ in the whole system. It labors under the order of the fiat of perfection. In short I will say that all parts are dependent upon the seed property of the blood when sent forth from the lungs to the heart and through the arterial system, the real system of delivery. We talk much about diseases and their causes; their deadly effects are from insufficient power of the body to recuperate.

We take up brain disease, diseases of the neck and spinal cord with the organs dependent on them for nerve force. We talk much and long which proves that the eye of the doctor closes before he realizes that some place in the body there must be a garden spot where the seed-like condition of the blood is developed. With this view I can talk to the practitioner and feel that I have a foundation. I can present the facts which will give the light necessary for the beginning philosopher. Ages have passed yet the people sicken, suffer, recover or die and by habit or tradition we still follow the unsuccessful practice and methods of the old theories.

A word to the doctor. I want you to open both eyes and look me square in the face. Can you afford in treating diseases of the lungs to give your verdict and prescribe drugs or manipulations as a doctor of medicine, an osteopath, or masseur, without first carefully examining the pleurae in all divisions and knowing that their nerve and blood supply are perfectly normal? In my opinion you are not warranted in making any move until you have found the condition of the pleura, the lung, the heart and all abdominal viscera and know that every variation of bone and muscle that would produce any suspension of nourishment to the pleura, heart, lungs or other organs of the system is found. Then you are warranted after a careful exploration in proceeding to adjust from the abnormal to the normal. Then you can expect the normal supply of both blood and nerve to all organs. Otherwise you will simply display your ability to give useless manipulations and show your ignorance of cause, and do little if any good for your patients.

If I have impressed the importance of the seedlike property of arterial blood, what I have said on this subject will do you good. If not, my time is lost and your work will be unsatisfactory in results both to your patient and yourself. Carefully read up the nerve and blood supply of the pleura, the nerve and blood supply of both lungs and the heart, because the lungs and the heart stand responsible for perfect health and every diseased organ depends on those two servants for recovery. Let us run over the machine beginning with the mouth which grinds the food. The food then passes into the throat, esophagus, stomach and the bowels where it is prepared to give and deliver the extract known as chyle. This is mixed with venous blood, taken to the heart, and from the heart it goes to the lungs or garden to be finished and returned to the heart as arterial blood, or seeds of animal life. Then it is sown through all parts of the body to sprout, grow and form bone, muscle, fiber and on to the sum total of all parts of the body.

FIND AND REMOVE THE CAUSE THEN THE EFFECT WILL DISAPPEAR.

All the organs of the system are subject to general laws of supply and action, and these laws extend to the parts of the system separately or combined; as much so as the earth is subject to the sunlight and darkness. During the hours of sunlight the earth receives the motor action from the sun and retains such substances as are necessary for animal and vegetable life. Then another condition called night takes the place of sunlight and all nature is benefited by it. The animal receives benefit from the common law of light and darkness; the vegetable and mineral receives from the same source that which is required by life for their growth. The relation of day and night to animal and vegetable growth shows the dependence of the earth upon the presence and absence of sunlight. The life of the whole globe would be a failure without the benefit of this one general law.

All organs and parts of the human body are the subjects of one general law of demand, supply, construction and renovation in order to keep up normal functioning. Our work as engineers then is to keep the engine so adjusted as to perform its functioning perfectly. Osteopathic adjustment means to so adjust the body that normal action will be sufficient to supply nerve force equal to the demand for construction, and to keep the body or organ in a healthy condition by casting out all impure substances before they become oppressive either from quantity or destructive and deadly poisonous chemical changes which result from stagnant fluids in the body. With this idea in view we are not at a loss to know how to proceed when we detect any cause that retains fluids that should have been passed on and out before such chemical action sets up.

We, as engineers, have but one question to ask—what has the body failed to do? If it is a failure in vision, hearing, smelling, tasting or motion of any part then it is the duty of the inspector to hunt for the cause that has produced the failure. In searching for the cause he should inquire of three witnesses, the nerves of sensation, motion and nutrition, for one or more has failed to perform its part in functioning. This law is just as absolute and indispensable to a healthy body as day and night are to the whole globe.

Should a failure occur in any part of the body, most any variation from normal urine will be found by urinalysis. This is an effect only, and to stop here as the world has done and still does, is no answer to an engineer's question—what and where is the cause of this confusion the result of which is sickness? I say this that you may follow me as an engineer. When you ask me why a lung, liver, kidney, uterus or bladder does not do its duty I want you to follow me to the excretory nerves of such organs. If you have given the proper attention to the nerve and blood supply to the heart, lung, liver, kidney, pleura, omentum, uterus or any other division of the body, you will know at once that the excretory nerves are overpowered at the point where they issue from the spinal cord, pneumogastric, solar plexus, or sympathetic; and without this knowledge your work will be a failure.

If by analysis you find that the urine has sugar, chalk, lime or any other impurities you have simply found the effect, and if you treat such effects successfully you must find the cause of friction, and proceed as a mechanic. Give your attention first to the sensory nerves to the kidney, heart or lung or other organ or limb of the body, then to the motor, excretory and nutrient nerves, for some of them are at fault and must be corrected. Then these nerves will soon dispose of all the bugaboos and microbes that have worried the doctor who treats effects. The man who is a competent engineer of the human body should not allow tumors to form and because of his lack of knowledge of cause and effect say that he does not know the cause of their production.

My object is to make the osteopath a philosopher, and place him on the rock of reason. Then I will not have the worry of writing details of how to treat any organ of the human body, because he is qualified to the degree of knowing what has produced variations of all kinds in form and motion. I want to establish in his mind the compass and searchlight by which to travel from the effect to the cause of all abnormality of the body. Then I will not have to detail what to do with misery in the head, on the face, with an aching heart, lung, pleura, liver, spleen, kidney or any organ or part of the body. He is right at home when he meets a tumor, because he knows and sees the cause and enters the combat, but not by any rule of special detailing, which belongs to the bunglesome book of symptomatology. When you fully comprehend and travel by the laws of reason, confusion will be a stranger in all your combats with disease.

PHILOSOPHY OF MANIPULATIONS.

The philosophy of manipulations is based upon an absolute knowledge of the form and function of all bones belonging to the bony framework of the human body. We must know the position and purpose of each bone and be thoroughly acquainted with each of its articulations. Without this knowledge our work will be a failure. Simply to know that our heads are situated upon the atlas and the atlas on the axis, that we have seven bones in the neck, twelve in the dorsal region and five in the lumbar is of little use. We must have a perfect image of the normal articulations of the bone or bones that we wish to adjust. We must be critically certain that we know all articulations of the bones of the whole system. We must know how the blood is supplied and when that arterial blood has done its work we must know how it returns and what would be an obstruction that would prevent its return. Without this information our opinion as to cause of variations from the perfectly healthy condition is without foundation, for our mechanical detection has failed to acquaint our minds with the cause that produces the abnormal condition in a perfectly healthy system. Thus a failure to give relief results in disappointment. The osteopathic mechanic must remember that Nature is a living critic and the answer must be yes or no. A normal image of the form and function of all parts of the body must be seen by the mind's eye or our work will condemn us.

Variations of the neck produce spasms in some persons, headache, dizziness and many other troubles in others. Strains, partial dislocations or other variations from a perfectly normal articulation of any of the lower four cervical or the upper four dorsal vertebrae have much if not all to do in producing shaking palsy of the head and arms, and a number of other diseases. From occiput to coccyx you must know right from wrong or the results will not give satisfaction. Now this is a very interesting subject and you must give it the most careful attention or you are not worthy of the confidence of the afflicted.

For thirty-five years I have labored to acquaint myself with the exact form of every bone that belongs to the framework of man's whole body. I have given attention not only to the form of each bone but also to why it is different in form and action from all other bones; to its exact location and articulation so that when it is removed from its place I know just where it belongs and how to take it and place it in the position that the builder intended for it. For days, months and years, and many of them, I have examined and criticised the normal and the abnormal position of all bones of the whole system. By this extensive study I have formed in my head a perpetual image of every articulation in the framework of the human body.

RELATION OF BONES TO DISEASES.

Without a thorough knowledge and long practice we make many blunders about what diseases follow injuries of the hip joint. I took up the thigh bone with its rounded head, and the socket in which Nature intended it should stay, and studied them for years. After critical examination I found that a dislocation of the head of the thigh bone from the socket would produce tightening of the muscles and flesh in that region and stop the venous return producing congestion, stagnation, fermentation and varicose veins of the whole limb from socket to sole of foot. I find that fermentation extends to the degree of inflammation; that the inflammatory process will extend from the hip joint to the occiput producing most all of the effects known as neuralgia, sciatica, lumbago, hardening and stiffening of the spine. I think I am talking to intellects who know the difference between fanciful words and demonstrated facts.

Is a bone personally responsible in performing any duty beyond its service as a brace or support for the body while in the erect position? Does its personality extend beyond that purpose? Is it a house in which a process of manufacturing substances for repairing takes place? Does it construct its own habitation? A thigh bone to all intents and purposes is a personality in receiving, repairing and constructing the bone directly from blood. We see that bone is filled with a substance ordinarily known as marrow or medullary substance; but in order to perform its duty as a functionary it must have blood to construct with, and all gates to the approach of blood must be opened. The entire length of the arterial course from the heart to the medullary substance of the thigh bone must be open or the result will be shrinkage of the flesh and starvation of the bone. If the arterial gates are open and the venous are closed, a variation from normal venous drainage results, and the detained venous blood becomes stagnant; stagnation means fermentation, inflammation and death to that substance or marrow. Then there forms an abscess with a discharge of this dead fluid made by stagnation and chemical action and decomposition of membranes.

As the thigh bone has openings or doors to receive arterial blood at the upper end, a partial or complete dislocation of the head of the femur from its socket would naturally shut off the blood supply. A dislocation of the femur produces a twist of the muscles around the neck of the bone putting the muscles and membranes on a stretch and producing pressure sufficient to shut off the nerve and blood supply to this bone. Then we have inflammatory rheumatism, and we are in possession of the knowledge of the cause that has produced this abnormality. Allow yourself to think of the nerve and blood supply to the acetabulum, innominates, sacrum and spine from the socket to the brain. Haven't you a cause equal to the production of renal calculi inflammation of the bones from the coccyx to the atlas with all the effects that follow spinal and sacral inflammation such as ossification of some or all of the joints of the spine? Do we not know that inflammatory yeast is the result of injuries and strains in the region of the head of the femur, and that the effects of this inflammatory fluid are as sure to travel up the spine as tetanus or lockjaw is to follow an injury to the foot caused by driving a large rusty nail through it?

I want the attention of an engineer because to him a fact is a truth. He reasons with ability. He always halts at the diseased points either of muscle or bone. He makes his conclusion as to the cause that has produced the abnormal condition from the cause of the friction which has produced adhesion of bone, decay of bone, inflammation and decay of flesh or whatever be the abnormality. To him the effect is a personality and he reasons that he must deal with the absolute truth or fail. He has abnormal variations to contend with and sees their effects from the crown of the head to the sole of the foot. To him knowledge is food and mental nourishment and theories are not what he wants. He wants the truth that is self-demonstrating and that stands upon the stone of eternal certainty. He cannot be guided by a dead compass. He reasons that when blood, urine and other fluids are diseased, there is a cause for it and that he can find it. He will hunt for and know where the friction is or tell you like an honest man that he does not know the cause.

MECHANICAL INSPECTION OR EXAMINATION.

It is expected that the mechanic will give a critical examination and a trustworthy report of such an examination. He has a square, a plumb and a level. By the square he ascertains the fact that all parts are in line, and any variation is told at once when the square is applied to the journal. With the level he ascertains whether all corners are on a level and equal. So far his foundation is square and level. He has one more witness—the plumb. It tells whether the superstructure stands perfectly erect or leans to one side or the other. He squares, plumbs and levels all foundations, journals and boxings. He examines all pulleys to know that they are in place and position. He examines the belt to see if one side is longer than the other. He corrects and goes on. He goes to the engine with the same instruments in his hand, inspects, squares, and levels the foundation that supports the engine. With the square and plumb he adjusts the drive wheels, pulleys and journals, then he inspects all pipes conducting water to his boiler and all pipes conducting steam to the chest. He examines safety and mud valves to know that they are ready to do normal work, then he inspects the furnace to know that here all is in proper order and in condition to throw the greatest amount of heat to the boiler. After making all corrections he fires up, starts the engine and if the answer is perfect work he knows that he has done his duty. For fear that something might give way he keeps his eye on the machinery for a few hours or days that he may feel satisfied that it is in good working order. He knows where and how the power is generated, how applied, and the uses of all the parts of the machinery.

Can an osteopath afford to ignore the sacred truth just illustrated by comparison when called upon to inspect, find and correct the cause of such friction as will result in imperfect action of the powers and principles of the human body? As a mechanic, I say no. His talk and work will prove him to be a dangerous person with whom to intrust the sacred work of life in all departments of the human body. This subject is too serious not to come under the most crucial and exact requirements of which human skill is master. If a mechanic is so particular to inspect every part and principle belonging to a steam engine for the purpose of getting good results, can you as an engineer omit any bone in the body and claim to be a trustworthy engineer? Can you say that any part has no importance physiologically, in this the greatest engine ever produced—the engine of human life? The operator is to remember the responsibility hanging over his head when he is in the sick room. You must reason, or fail. A hint to the wise is enough. I have given you a compass that will guide you out of many dark places. This is as old as all ages and as trustworthy in the hands of an osteopath as multiplication is to the mathematician. I want to emphasize to the student or operator the absolute unqualified importance of knowing the duties and personal responsibilities of a bone in keeping up its part as a laboratory and building.

VARIATION AND ADJUSTMENT
OF BONES.

As I am talking to mechanics who have a comprehensive knowledge of the human body and all of its machinery, powers, principles and motions, I shall talk in plain English. The mother language is the only language in which we can successfully think. We say head, neck, skull, bone, jaw, back bone, ribs, collar bone, shoulder blades, hip bones, thigh bones, shin bones, bones of the feet, bones of the arm, bones of the hand, and so on.

Now I will talk to you about bones. If you are an American you do not know what "os" is because it is out of your language. When I say "os" or "osseous system" you do not think "bones" at once. I will say muscle, skin, hair, and when I talk English to you and tell you to go and adjust an abnormal condition, if you understand your anatomy, I am not disappointed when I inspect your work.

If the normal position and relation of every bone from the crown of the head to the sole of the foot is a condition necessary to good health, what variation from a socket, facet or any joint will be the cause of some progressive disease such as a fever, tuberculosis, or inflammation of any joint of the neck, back, loin, hip, legs or arm? Can you as an engineer reconciled to your knowledge of a twist of a bone from its normal position, not see that such a slight movement would carry a muscle, both ends of which are fastened, backwards or forwards sufficiently far to produce an unnatural crossing of those fibrinous strings, muscles or tendons that unite a rib with the spinous process, or that unite other parts? Don't you see that in this condition there is a great strain and irritation at the point where one muscle crosses another? Don't you reason that normal vital action is suspended from this point back to the spinal cord or ganglion from which the nerve of this muscle is sent off, and beyond this point this vital action is a failure? As an engineer you see friction, as a philosopher you conclude there is an obstruction, and as a mechanic you remove the obstruction by so adjusting the bones that no strain is on a muscle causing it to press on another muscle, blood-vessel, ligament or nerve.

When you are combating effects such as diseases of the scalp, brain, eye, ear, tongue, throat, lung, heart, liver, spleen, pancreas, stomach, bowels, kidneys, bladder, womb, or limbs you will arrive at a trustworthy conclusion as to cause if you use the method of reasoning just outlined. There is no part that I have named which if affected by disease does not present a philosophical question to be answered by an engineer and not by an imitator nor a masseur. The friction or cause that has produced the disease must be removed and normality established. An honest, thoroughbred, well-qualified engineer knows by his qualification and experience that each variation from normal action in an engine has a definite cause, and the friction of a pulley should never be treated at the steam chest. He must have the power of reason to hold perpetually before his eyes a perfectly normal image of any part of the human bony system, then he can judge just what is the cause of the malady he has to contend with.

Here is a list of leading questions to ask the mechanical critic, the philosopher and the engineer who can reason from the effect or friction to the cause producing such effect. Why do one person's eyes when congested become abnormally large and a constant stream of tears pass from them? Where is the friction responsible for this unnatural appearance of the eye? Would you go to the nerve and blood supply of the eye for the cause or would you cut those eyes out and throw them away? If you have polyps or adenoid tumors of the nose, would you take the tongs and pull out some nose this month and some more nose every other month or would you go to the nerve and blood supply and the drainage and regulate them? If you were consulted on a case of enlarged tonsils would you take your knife out of your belt, whack them off and throw them away or would you go to the atlas and axis as a sensible engineer, and give Nature a chance to reduce the tonsil to its normal condition? You must know first, last and all the time that if the blood could have passed to and from the head without obstruction there would be no tumor.

Suppose there should be inflammation and soreness of the trachea and esophagus, would an engineer account for the friction by imperfect blood and nerve action or would he swab the throat with destructive caustic and other poisons? Would an osteopath accept such conclusion or action as a truth or would he book such procedure as ignorance of cause and effect? Suppose an engineer who knows his business is consulted on what is known as pleuro-pneumonia, and the lungs are laboring under much excitement and congestion. Would that engineer fire up with hot water bags, administer morphine, whiskey, digitalis, strychnine, or would he explore the spine and ribs from the diaphragm to the head for slips, strains, and dislocations of the bones of the spine to know why this shut-off from the blood and nerve supply and to know why the pneumogastric could not do its normal work and allow the blood to pass to and from the brain, pleura and lungs?

An engineer who knows his business does not hesitate to proceed at once to adjust all parts of the neck, and passing down from the head and neck he adjusts all parts to the dorsal. Would he be satisfied to stop his work without knowing to a certainty that the clavicular articulation is absolutely correct or would he leave the clavicle sufficiently far back off the acromian process to shut off the jugular vein so that it could not deliver venous blood to the heart? He knows that he is dealing with a train that is running very fast, and from the condition of the road it will soon be ditched if he does not adjust his engine and do it very quickly. His object is perfect drainage from head, face, neck, pleura, lung, intercostals and all parts of the thoracic division. He knows that when all pressure is removed from the pneumogastric, harmony will follow in its action; that when the resistance caused by closure at the point where the ascending carotid enters the head is taken off, the unnecessary labors of the arterial system will stop because the veins or mud valves are doing trustworthy work. Then breathing and heart action become normal. Relief and recovery are sure to follow if the engineer knows and does his work.

Mr. Engineer, allow me to ask you a few more questions that I think are of the greatest importance to the success of the science of osteopathy. I have asked you questions in reference to the head, face, eyes, neck and organs of the thorax and I think you are worthy and well qualified to take charge and safely run this engine so far as the organs above the diaphragm are concerned. Now a few hasty questions in reference to the liver. When the nerve and blood supply to this important organ are good, is that all that is necessary for it to do good work? You say "yes, give me nerve force, blood supply, drainage, and plenty of nourishing diet and I will guarantee the results to be good and satisfactory." Suppose there should be enlargement of the liver, what conclusion would you came to? I would say at once if there is no mechanical injury to contend with that a failure of the venous drainage causes this congestion and overgrowth: Would you suggest purgatives, stimulants, dietetics, going to the mountains, pukes, blisters and hot bags? I would not, I would explore the nerve and blood supply and drainage of the whole hepatic system. I would correct all bony abnormalities, give my patient rest, plenty of good wholesome food and expect to soon have a liver normal in all particulars, provided I am called in reasonable time and the patient is not exhausted and disabled from poisonous drugs. The same rule is just as good and trustworthy in diseases of the spleen, pancreas, stomach, bowels, kidneys, uterus, bladder and limbs.

One asks, "how must we pull a bone to replace it"? I reply, pull it to its proper place and leave it there. One man advises you to pull all bones you attempt to set until they "pop." That "popping" is no criterion to go by. Bones do not always "pop" when they go back to their proper places nor does it mean they are properly adjusted when they do "pop". If you pull your finger you will hear a sudden noise. The sudden and forceable separation of the ends of the bones that form the joint causes a vacuum and the air entering from about the joint to fill the vacuum causes the explosive noise. That is all there is to the "popping" which is fraught with such significance to the patient who considers the attempts at adjustment have proven effectual. The osteopath should not encourage this idea in his patient as showing something accomplished.

Another asks, "how do you set a hip or any other dislocation, partial or complete"? You have asked a big question which requires a correct answer. Previous to readjusting any bone of the body, it matters not which one it is or how far it has been forced from its socket, you must first loosen it at its attachments at its articulating end, always bearing in mind that when a bone has left its proper articulation the surrounding muscles and ligaments are irritated and keep up a continual contracture.

We have a thigh bone out of its socket and pressed very closely to a point on the surface of the ilium. Bend the knee very slightly, place one hand under the foot and the other hand under the trochanter major; with the hand at the foot while the leg is bent, push knee up towards patient's face put your chest or chin against the knee and with the hand under the foot pull towards you and with chin or chest push knee from you. At this time the head of the femur has been pressed or twisted out from the ilium. Now with the hand at the trochanter you have head of the femur within range of its socket, so bring the lame leg over and across the knee of the well leg; pull down slightly on the foot and as you take the lame leg off the sound knee straighten the leg out and the hip is set without a "pop" or pain, as the hand under the trochanter major has suspended sensation in the limb. This is one of many methods of setting a hip. Without going into detail further I will say that all dislocations, partial or complete, can be adjusted by this rule First loosen the dislocated end from other tissues, then gently bring it back to its original place.

In setting a shoulder, after a thorough loosening at the articulation, use but little force to push the elbow towards the contracted muscles at the shoulder then rotate the humerus into its socket.

I will say to the student of osteopathy, to judges, jurors, lawyers and all interested, that there are many ways to set bones; there are many ways to bring them from their abnormal position back to their normal articulation. In adjusting bones the mechanic is governed by three principles—the lever, the screw and the wedge. To remove a bone or any substance from its position the mechanic seeks to find and make a fixed point then he makes use of the principle of the lever, the screw or the wedge and with his hands gets the movement desired.

A partial or complete dislocation of any bone becomes a weight or resisting power. The hand or any other substance may be used as a fulcrum. Then the rib, femur or any other bone becomes your lever, and by applying your power outside of the fulcrum the weight or resistance can be overcome.

I am often asked how I would adjust the spine or ribs in asthma, in lung and heart trouble. In cases of asthma one of my methods is to place my patient's back against the door-facing. The door makes a fixed point against the back and holds it firmly in position. With my fingers on the rib or ribs that are above or below the articulation with the transverse process, I take the arm back and up with considerable force. This movement of the arm is to put the serratus magnus muscle on that side on a strain which helps to draw the rib up. After holding my hand firmly against the rib while the arm is in that position I swing the arm back and down.

Another method I use is to place my patient on his back on the table and bring the arm on the affected side out at a right angle. Then I place my thigh close up in the axillary region and push the arm upward putting the serratus magnus on a strain as before. At the same time I pass my hand back of the shoulder and place my fingers on the affected rib and push up or down as the case may require. These are two methods, but there are many more that I think are just as good.

I want to make it plain that there are many ways of adjusting bones. And when one operator does not use the same method as another, it does not show criminal ignorance on the part of either, but simply the getting of results in a different manner. A skilled mechanic has many methods by which he can produce the desired result. A fixed point, a lever, a twist, or a screw power, can be and are used by all operators. The choice of methods is a matter to be decided by each operator and depends on his own skill and judgment. One operator is right handed, the other left. They will choose different methods to accomplish the same thing. Every operator should use his own judgment and choose his own method of adjusting all bones of the body. It is not a matter of imitation and doing just as some successful operator does, but the bringing of the bone from the abnormal to the normal.

SOME MECHANICAL INJURIES AND THEIR EFFECTS.

A wound or injury, when sufficiently severe, will produce sudden death. A gun-shot wound or a wound with a knife or bayonet often produces instantaneous death because of the magnitude of the nervous shock. This truth is very evident when the wound is in the brain, because the whole nervous system depends upon the brain for force and nourishment. When a knife or bullet passes through a chamber of the heart and spills the blood out it is certain to produce death, for we have a perverted action, a stoppage of the arterial blood flow. We have death from shock to the nervous system which has been depleted by loss of blood.

So far we have been dealing with wounds centrally located. Now we will change the location of wounds placing them in the flesh of a finger, hand or arm. These by their progressive action reach the two centers or seats of life, the brain and the heart. They may result in a shock to the nervous system producing tetanus and death. The poisonous venom of a snake inserted into the opening made by the tooth of the serpent in many cases progresses with its irritation to the nervous system until death is the result. Often a broken toe or finger results in erysipelas, blood poison and death. These injuries are visible and we know the results. Suppose we note a few invisible injuries such as occur about the hip joint.

When a hip is thrown out of the socket, and tears, strains or wounds the tissues, muscles and nerves, and inhibits the normal action of blood, is it at all surprising to say that this accounts for many diseases that have baffled the skill of the medical world for all ages, such as hysteria, confused menstruation, constipation, bladder and kidney disease, and on up as high as the liver and spleen, where is located the great solar plexus, the center of nerve distribution of the abdomen? This wound of the hip travels far back to the solar plexus producing inhibition of the nutrient branches passing from the solar plexus to the lung, spleen, stomach and all organs of the abdomen and pelvis sufficient to produce an unhealthy condition of these organs. Now can we expect the heart and lungs to produce good healthy blood from the chyle produced by the wounded organs of the abdomen, omentum, and peritoneum? I think not.

From my experience I think that much of the disease to which men and women are subject is the result of an injury about the hip joint. I think I have detailed enough of the effect produced by an abnormal hip on the nervous system and back to the solar plexus to prove to any person reasoning from effect to cause that he should never leave a patient with the hip and pelvic articulation unexplored. We have relieved constipation, uterine hemorrhage and bladder trouble by adjusting the head of the thigh bone, the innominates and the sacrum. There has been too little attention given to shocks and injuries to the muscles and nerves about the hip joints, and I think here lies the reason for so much uncomprehended truth concerning the diseases of this region of the body. We as anatomists and physiologists should record the truths learned from our experience, for the reading and consideration of future generations. I want the osteopaths to raise the flag of reason and fight for victory over such diseases as above named.

Having a thorough knowledge of the descriptive anatomy and diseases of the bones—of the lumbar vertebrae, of the sacrum, of the innominates and the femur—an osteopath reasons that dislocations of one or both femurs from the socket, whether much or little, or bruises or strains at the hip, result in inhibition producing such diseases. In persons suffering from hysteria, constipation, womb or bladder troubles and many other diseases, I have found a looseness at and around the acetabulum indicating a ligation of the nerve and blood supply as it passes to and from the thigh bone. To retain venous blood in the medullary substance in a femur produces congestion, stagnation and neuralgic manifestations all the way from the acetabulum to the dorsal vertebrae. The solar plexus throws its branches in great numbers from the crura to the coccyx and it is reasonable and undisputable that confusion and disease, such as paralysis of the lower bowels, and nerve and blood supply of the uterus, may be expected to follow such injuries. Then we may expect nerve irritation periodically which carries on its convulsive or spasmodic action known as hysteria and various other abdominal and pelvic disorders.

I would advise the osteopathic practitioner to keep posted on descriptive anatomy and physiology from surgical writers on diseases of bones in order to know that he is in the proper location to find the cause of this multitude of diseases. The bones and muscles from the lumbar vertebrae to the knee are subject to high inflammation, decomposition and sloughing away, and the philosophy following in this line of thought concerning the cause of such effects (as these diseases) has never before, so far as we know, been pointed out by any writer. Since giving my attention to this subject for the last thirty years I have been troubled but little as to the origin and cause of such effects. If you expect to be a successful mechanic, act like one who is governed by the square, plumb and level of reason, knowing just why such effects have been produced.

We see a great many cases, and read of others, that are diagnosed and demonstrated as congenital dislocations of the hip. Ask the surgeon to tell you what he means by congenital dislocation of the hip and what is the cause. Read all authorities to the present date to see what information you can obtain as to the cause of these conditions described as congenital dislocation. When you have faithfully listened as a mechanic to the whole story you are left without a word that points to the cause of such a condition.

Suppose we call it nurse's disease of the hip, and when we talk to a mechanic tell him that there has been enough cloth piled between the child's legs to make a fulcrum upon which the thigh bone has been used as a lever, when she pinned the cloth and by her strong hands brought the legs together. With the cloth as a fulcrum and the thigh bone as a lever she has in this way pried both hips out of the socket. If there is anything congenital about this condition it is ignorance of this effect. The mother and the nurse should know that bringing the knees together over this rag fulcrum would pry both hips out of the sockets. When will the doctor advise that a child's limbs must be let loose in order to be healthy?

I will emphasize as a mechanic that he who reasons will see at once the importance of hunting for all causes, both great and small, that would produce shocks of the nervous system; for such shocks are followed by confusion in the physiological laboratory of animal life. So small a thing as a pin, nail or thorn driven into the body sometimes produces a shock that is followed by suspended nerve action and stoppage of the blood in its venous circulation from the extremities back to the heart and lungs. A jolt that would produce a slip of a rib enough to cause contraction of a fiber of muscle or ligament would produce an irritation that would detain the blood long enough to ferment and produce erysipelas with all its deadly effects. Thus the importance of never stopping until you have found the cause producing abnormal effects designated by such names as diphtheria, scarlet fever, pneumonia, pleurisy and all other abnormal variations of the head, neck, thorax, abdomen and pelvis.

We must comprehend the importance and magnitude of a wound, and the poisons that come from stagnation and fermentation. If we inject morphine into the foot it is soon taken up by the nervous system and becomes a universal poison. The bite of a snake or a mad dog, or gas inhaled into the lungs is taken up and distributed through the body at once and death follows. My object is to emphasize the importance of looking after local causes that go on with their irritation. A slip of the under jaw or neck causes facial paralysis, facial neuralgia, or if you prefer the term, tic douloureux. Such diseases as shaking palsy, smallpox, measles, mumps, chickenpox, diphtheria, enlarged tonsils, adenoid tumors, dysentery, constipation, bloody flux, monthly irregularities or any variation from health have a cause, and the cause has a location. It is the business of the osteopath to locate and remove it doing away with the disease and getting health instead. I want the osteopath to be a hunter and find his game, otherwise his work will be unsatisfactory.

REGION OF THE HEAD

REGION OF THE HEAD.

In my classification in this book my object has been to give a system of exploration for the cause of disease, and for its treatment according to the location, blood and nerve supply of the affected part. I begin with the head as I consider it the organ or division of the body in which most of the nerve fluid and force for the use of the entire body is generated and stored. The body constitutes the shop in which all substances pertaining to the physical makeup are manufactured. I say all, I mean all, and I mean it all the time when I am talking to the practical operator.

The head is as much dependent on the lung, the heart and all organs below as they are on the head. Without such interdependence the organs of the five senses would in all reason be failures. Because of this interdependence I want to insist on bringing to your attention the importance in treating diseases of the head, of keeping the road from the heart to the brain open and in first class condition for the passage and delivery of pure arterial blood to the head. The free and unobstructed return of the venous blood is just as important. This law is exact and absolute and if you want perfect hearing, vision, smell, taste, feeling, you must have good nourishment, pure abundant arterial blood, nerve fluid, and an open way for venous return.

Now with this fact before you, together with your knowledge of the human machinery and its physiological duties in life, you have a foundation upon which to reason, and a guide to direct you in your search for causes which produce effects in this division of the body.

When we are consulted on baldness, dandruff and skin diseases of the head we are constrained to ask these questions: Is the arterial supply normal? Is the venous drainage normal? Our conclusion is, that this falling hair is an effect, the result of either imperfect arterial supply or venous drainage, and that the debris or dandruff is the substance that should have been used for the growth and health of the hair. The abnormality of blood and nerve supply and venous drainage is the cause that has produced this effect.

Any bone removed from its normal position in the neck or chest, be that posterior, anterior or lateral, is obstruction enough to produce a pressure on the vertebral or carotid arteries and interfere with the normal blood supply.

Then we reason that this abnormality is the cause of a disturbance of the harmonious action of the brain itself because of the shortage of blood produced by such impingement. Not only would the bones obstruct but the muscles of the neck becoming irritated and contractured produce suspension of the normal flow of blood to and from the brain.

THE BRAIN AS A STOREHOUSE.

All physiologists agree that a qualified system of nerves pass from the brain to each part of the body, be that part skin, fascia, tissue, bone, bowel, liver, heart or lung; every part must have power in proportion to its needs in carrying out its individual work. Then we know the brain to be the storehouse supplying all organs, and all roads and gates leading to or coming from it must be open all the time or confusion will be the condition and show effects which according to some rule are given names.

Now our work is to open wide all the gates and turn in the blood to each and every organ. They will do the rest. Keep these organs supplied with nerve force and blood in order that they may keep their work of construction up to the normal standard. This cannot be done when by inhibition, pressure, or any other cause, the nerve force falls below the normal demand. A destroyed or severed nerve can do just as much good as a nerve whose power is totally inhibited. It is wholly useless to present reasons why a thing is or is not the effect of such causes. For this reason I try to assist the osteopathic operator to realize that he must know what to do and how to do it.

If a locomotive engineer turns on the steam and it fails to be received into and discharged from the cylinders and he does not have enough skill about him to find the cause of the inhibition, he would soon find himself discharged as an incompetent and dangerous man in the position, because the safety and the lives of all persons on the train depend on the engineer's knowledge of his business. Now when any or all of the organs of the body are in a disturbed condition the engineer must find the exact place where the "steam of life" is cut off or the entire train or organs will be thrown off their track.

To apply this thought we will say that the blood, or the "steam of life" leaves the heart, passes up the neck to be delivered to and supply the brain, but meets with inhibition just before it enters the skull. Would an engineer reason that no bad effect would follow such inhibition? If he knew nothing about the parts and principles of the engine he would say, "great is the mystery of why tumefactions appear in the nose, ear, tonsils, submaxillary and thyroid glands; great is the mystery of congestion of the lungs," and so on. All of which any competent osteopathic engineer would reason about and conclude that he must remove the obstruction which exists to the normal flow of blood from start to destination.

It matters not what the talkist says about microorganisms. No matter how much laboratory experience he marshals and talks wisely about, he must let that blood find its unobstructed way to its destination or else his suffering patient will die.

DISEASES OF THE SCALP.

Etiology.—I have always attributed such abnormalities as dandruff, falling off of the hair, lumpy growths or cysts to a shortage in the nerve supply, obstruction of proper blood circulation and the drainage of both the venous and lymphatic systems of the superficial fascia.

In all cases of baldness or dandruff which I have examined and successfully treated I have found the atlas or axis in one of four positions; either to the right, left, front or rear, hence abnormal. I have reasoned and worked for good circulation of all the fluids in the superficial fascia of the entire head and face and have gotten good results (particularly so for men) in such cases as were not of too long standing.

Treatment.—I begin my work with the atlas and extend my treatment to all the bones, muscles and ligaments as low down as the eighth dorsal. I correct all malpositions of bones. In order to get a good supply of nourishment I adjust them all from the atlas to the diaphragm. To loosen up all the muscles in this spinal area I bring my thumbs on both sides of the neck with strong pressure as they glide down over the muscles of the neck to about the fourth dorsal.

Wash the scalp, then oil it with some animal oil such as neat's-foot oil or lard. I oil the scalp thoroughly then with a coarse cloth I rub it vigorously to loosen up the skin, fascia and muscles in order to give room for a good vigorous circulation of blood, nerve and lymphatic fluids. Use a coarse cloth to take off all surplus grease. This I do about once a week for a few times. In many cases I have had the hair return to its normal condition.

When I find a scalp with cysts I give such patients the benefit of surgery laying the scalp open and taking out the entire cyst. On some heads I have found a half dozen or more. I simply split the skin open, take the sac out, bring the edges together. I never found it necessary to stitch up the opening but place a small cloth over it and press it down into the blood. This cloth need not be over one inch in width. I let it remain until the union of the edges has become complete.

This has been my procedure with cysts; but as they belong to the department of osteopathic surgery I would advise you to treat all such abnormal growths of the scalp accordingly. There may be aneurysms and various other conditions to deal with which require the advice, experience and skill of a practicing surgeon. I would advise those of you who have not taken the surgical course to call an osteopath who has.

ERUPTIONS OF THE FACE.

Etiology.—All eruptions of the face such as pimples, which are very common to young men and women, are simply effects of imperfect action of the nerve and blood supply to the skin.

Treatment.—This condition I have found could be relieved by obtaining healthy circulation of the fluids of the nerves and vessels of the superficial fascia of the face and head. I obtain this when I have a properly adjusted atlas, axis and all of the bones of the neck. I am very particular to know that the blood not only goes to the brain and does its work there, but goes also to the fascia and skin, and that the return of the venous blood is absolutely normal.

After adjusting the bones and muscles of the neck I loosen up and proceed to knead the musculature of the neck with my thumbs, using a gliding motion, because I want the blood and all the fluids to have perfect circulation and nourish normally the bones, muscles, fascia and the skin.

DISEASES OF THE EYE.

General Discussion.—In dealing with the eye you want to note the deep and superficial effects and travel to the cause. The osteopath must reason by the principles of philosophy that will guide him in a thorough search for the cause that has produced the condition with which he has to contend. The first question that arises in the mind of the osteopath is: Is the nerve and blood supply normal? When found in an abnormal condition (surgical injuries excepted) he must first take up the form and function, and acquaint himself with the nerve and blood supply. Then he is prepared to search for and know what would cause a stoppage in blood supply, drainage and the nerve forces used in the whole process of construction, motion, use and nourishment of all parts and principles belonging to the motion and use of the eye.

Etiology and Examination.—By all methods of reason he is forced to establish the heart as his foundation or starting point, as the blood and nerve supply must both work in perfect harmony. Go from the heart upwards and explore the carotid arteries and the bones of the neck and upper dorsal and know that every joint from the atlas to the fourth dorsal is correct. If so, examine and see that the upper ribs, the dorsal vertebrae and the clavicles are truly normal in position. If not, you are not warranted to leave this field of examination until you correct the atlas and all bones in the cervical and upper dorsal region because the nerves in this region will fail to do proper functioning if not well supplied with force from the brain and with blood direct from the heart. Then it is just as important that when this blood has done its work it shall be returned to the heart without delay.

Here I have given you all the instruction that I think is necessary to hunt and know the cause that produces cataract, dripping eyes and all other eye failures or variations from normal work, because no failure in nerve or blood supply can be tolerated and have the eye in condition to perform such duties as are designed for that organ. Here is a list of various diseases of the eye which come directly under the guidance of this philosophy: Lachrymosis, pterygium, granulated lids, astigmatism, strabismus and cataract.

TREATMENT.

Lachrymation.—In lachrymation, or dripping eyes, I have succeeded in stopping the weeping or dripping by adjusting the axis with the atlas. Sometimes I have treated as low as the fifth cervical producing a complete cure.

Pterygium.—I have treated many cases of pterygium, removing the growth and leaving the eye in its original condition. In all cases of pterygium I go to the nasal bones which you know are situated just a little below the bridge of the nose where the spectacles cross the nose. I place my thumbs on both sides of the nose on the upper part of the nasal bones and gently but firmly push the nasal bones down towards the eye teeth. I do this in order to get a free circulation of the fluids and let them pass out of the pterygium. By so doing I have succeeded in removing them. In a few weeks, two to four, the pterygium has generally passed away under the treatment just indicated.

Granulated Lids.—For granulated lids I treat the nasal bones just about the same as I would for pterygium. I carefully examine the neck and adjust all variations from the normal. Beginning with the atlas I carefully explore as low down as the second rib and correct all abnormal conditions found; then, with the finger nail carefully trimmed so it will not irritate the lid, and the finger softened with warm water, insert the index finger tip under the lid and pass from side to side. It would be well enough to oil the finger with vaseline, milk or any soft oil so as not to irritate the lid. After stretching the lid moderately I found this to be about all that was necessary for granulated lids and purulent sore eyes. The results have been perfectly satisfactory to me as well as to the patients.

Astigmatism.—In what is generally known as astigmatism I address my treatment along the whole extent of the neck from the atlas to the sixth cervical. I am very particular to adjust the facets of the fifth to those of the sixth cervical in order to give nourishment to the eye, the lack of which I think is the cause of astigmatism. If the eye has not been injured by drugs I have succeeded in relieving that feeble condition called astigmatism and in returning the eye to its normal functioning.

Strabismus.—We have straightened out a great many eyes by adjusting the neck very carefully from the atlas to the first dorsal, particularly the articulation of the fifth cervical with the sixth. Cases of long standing may be surgical.

CATARACT.

Etiology.—We see that light brought to a focus by a double convex lens produces great heat. We can use the light of the sun to burn wood, coal, melt metals, glass, etc. Now we find in the eye a well formed double convex crystalline lens that is so powerful in condensing the rays of the sun-light that the eye would be ruined by the heat thus condensed if continued for a long period.

I want to draw your attention to the atomizing power of light. We have reason to know that the crystalline lens condenses or focalizes light in the eye-chamber strong enough to atomize opaque bodies and a failure of the lens to produce this effect allows substances to be retained until they become bulky, opaque and obstructive to the nerves of vision. I think the failure of the crystalline lens to focalize light, and produce the gaseous condition of lymph and other substances that should be passed out while in this gaseous condition, is the cause producing cataracts. To me this is an established truth, established by experience and observation.

Treatment.—Adjust the bones of the upper spine, ribs and neck and re-establish normal nerve and blood supply. Then make a gentle tapping of the eye to loosen the crystalline lens a little. With one finger give a few flips or gentle taps on the back of another finger the soft part of which is held against the side of the eye. This tapping should be just strong enough to make the eye ache a little. Without any surgical interference whatever I have been rewarded in a majority of cases by the disappearance of that white substance in the eye called a cataract.

Remember when you are treating an eye for cataract that no rough treatment is expected to be administered to so delicate an organ. I have given you my experience for the consideration of the expert anatomical physiologist as he has the philosophy by which I have been governed when-I wished to dispose of opaque bodies. I have never given such treatments oftener than twice the first week and once a week thereafter, because the eye must have time to re-establish normal nerve and blood supply in order to obtain the results desired.

The operator will find that most or all of the variations of the eye from the normal condition are attributable to lesions found in the neck and upper dorsal region and will yield readily to proper adjustment of those parts.

I have been a little lengthy in the treatment of these diseases of the eye in order to encourage the operator to a thorough and careful examination of the neck and spine, because for many years I have been convinced that most all of the eye troubles are simply effects of failure in the nerve and blood supply. I think the operator will be rewarded with good results if he will confine himself to the structure of the neck and to re-establishing the nerve and blood supply, because on this foundation the osteopath's success depends.

REGION OF THE THROAT
AND NECK

DISEASES OF THROAT AND NECK.

In presenting to the student the subject of sore tonsils, diphtheria, scarlet fever, mumps and the various forms of throat and glandular diseases of the neck we feel that we would be placed in a very embarrassing position if we were to be guided by the writings or books that are called authority on such diseases. No two of them have agreed upon the diagnosis or treatment, or at least they have not established a reliable method that will guide you to a successful treatment in any of these diseases.

They fail to give us a philosophy regarding the cause of the incipient congestion, fermentation and on to the inflammation and sloughing away of the lining membranes and flesh of the mouth, throat, submaxillary and cervical glands. They simply assert that thus and so is tonsillitis, diphtheria, scarlet fever, mumps and so on through the list of names applied to such diseases as are confined to the cervical region, esophagus and trachea. I have perused book after book claimed to be standard authority on such diseases. They talk of analyzing the sputum and they tell us all about bacteria, all about the contagious nature of bacteria such as are found in the mucous membrane and glands of the neck, submaxillary and so on. So far we are just as blank as though we had not read the books nor analyzed the sputum and other substances. The patient is sick, suffering and dying, and we know this to be the condition. We call in counsel, trying to select the brightest lights of the day; and at the conclusion when we hoped light would appear we are let down into the dark mists of despair, for our patient is dead. We have received nothing.

This has been my experience for over fifty years. My money has been spent for books. My time has been lost in reading from the hundreds of authors I have consulted on diseases of the throat and neck and today the treatment is the same old story, quiet, opiates, apply liniments, swab with caustic, and with a pencil cut off the white covering found on different parts of the throat and tonsil. Our patient dies and all we can say is that from the observations of all doctors from the past up to the present time he has had the best scientific attention obtainable. We analyze the urine, we analyze the blood, we analyze the fecal matter, and we report the kinds and quantity of bacteria and the death of our patient.

Question: Is it not time that the osteopathic anatomists and physiologists lay down these old books that contain nothing but compilations of many thousands of pages of useless, and allow me to say senseless, speculative nonsense? Notwithstanding, many persons who seem to be well educated will practice according to those old theories. I say they practice today, and talk with as much vehemence as though they had a truth, but when applied, death is the verdict. Such men, to me are something like a mule born in a coal pit. His birth was in darkness and he has no concept of the meaning of the word light. We have just such mules today who can write all the big words and little words that mysticism has been able to produce and compile in a thousand centuries. They talk long and loud and sell us their voluminous works. We peruse them to the dead hour of midnight, waste our oil and physical energies and exclaim when through, "sold again!"

It is now left for the osteopath to collect all these old books and compilations, burn them up and throw them to the wind from whence they came. Let their ashes return to the earth as a fertilizer of the soil, for they have given no information by which the human mind has grown to useful intelligence. Let us be merciful to the old doctor. He has done the best he could but he has given us nothing. Let us say we admire his grit, but we cannot say the products handed down to us by the doctors of all ages give us an iota of that which we have sought—truth—that we can apply to our suffering patients and know from the beginning that the result will be re-establishment of health. We as osteopaths have raised the lone star of the mechanic. It has been up in open view for over thirty-five years and has established beyond all controversy that blood is the food of life. When the system can use it normally health is your answer; when not, disease and death are the words of your soliloquy.

You know that when water or any other liquid is spilling out of a barrel at what is generally called the bung-hole, if you drive a tight fitting cork into that hole no more liquid will leak out of it. I want to make the application direct to your mechanical thought so I will say the heart is the barrel and we will start a current of blood up from the heart to the brain and call the openings at the base of the skull where the arteries enter the head the bung-holes. Then the foramina through which the veins pass as they carry the blood back to the heart will also be called bung-holes.

Now don't you know that if the vein bung-holes are shut up, the heart will pump enough blood into the head to produce congestion of the brain? On the other hand, when we find the arterial bung-hole stopped up the heart continues to pump up the blood. As soon as one stroke stops another follows. There is no cessation there. If this arterial blood cannot get through that bung-hole it will overflow into the surrounding tissue and organs and deposit more than a normal quantity of blood in some place between the heart and bung hole, commencing at the base of the skull to make its deposits. As a result of this you will have enlarged glands which have received some of this arterial blood. The heart pumps away until this locality refuses to take any more blood, then you have congestion, stagnation, inflammation, chills, fever and all the symptoms that would accompany such conditions.

Suppose because of a change of weather, contracted muscles should close the bung-hole, then you have cause for tonsillitis and inflammation of the glands below the skull, in the neck and also in the mouth. You know well enough that the heart will pound away even when the tonsils, larynx or pharynx are crowded full of arterial blood which should pass on. This is a cause for inflammation in this region, and it is usually accompanied by congestion and inflammation of the deep and superficial glandular system of the neck including the thyroid and all of the glands, large and small, above the thorax.

I have given you a homely illustration, one such as might be given to a boy—which you are, if you have not attained to this knowledge. When your mind has comprehended the facts that I have just given you, the mystery of glandular disease of the neck, face and head becomes a practical philosophy to guide you in your explorations, treatment and care of such diseases. If you wish to correct these conditions, pull the bung out and let the blood flow on uninterruptedly from the heart which I have here represented as a barrel. I simply tell you that which I know and that which during years of experience I have demonstrated to myself to be Nature's only reliable remedy.

Now I will draw your attention to the successful treatment of the submaxillary glands which you will be consulted about very often during your practice. Venous blood is often retained in such a quantity as to set up an inflammatory irritation of the glands of the neck, which goes on and forms pus. This you will let out with your lance. Many other lumps will be found on one or both sides of the neck from the atlas to the seventh cervical. You will mentally ask the question, how is the blood stopped? This blood was sent up from the subclavian artery the whole length of the neck to the brain. When it has done its work it is reasonable that it should be returned to the heart for renewal. Should it fail to return from those glands inflammation will follow to the degree of forming pus. Your work is to lift the clavicles and adjust the ribs so that the venous blood is not obstructed on its way through the vena cava back to the heart. As you are well versed in anatomy and physiology, I feel a little timid about insisting on the perfect freedom of the arteries that supply, and the veins that drain the glandular system of the neck. But the demand for their freedom is absolute and we must be governed accordingly. A sore tongue, sore eyes, sore tonsil, sore nose, running ears, the nasal air passages and all the membranes rapidly heal when you have secured perfect drainage.

LARYNGEAL DISEASES.

Definition of Laryngitis.—Inflammation of the larynx; inflammation of the mucous membrane of the larynx. Simple catarrhal laryngitis in some measure resembles croup, but is usually devoid of the peculiar sonorous inspiration of the latter. There is pain upon pressing the larynx, and while laryngitis is a disease of more advanced life, croup attacks children. Membraniform exudation is also absent, probably because the inflammation being seated above the glottis, the coagulable lymph is readily expectorated. It requires the most active treatment.

—Dunglison.

Etiology.—In considering the cause or causes of laryngitis in any or all forms, I reason that it is an effect and we now wish to ascertain the cause of such effect. This division or organ of the body is situated on the front side of the neck and receives its blood supply from the superior and inferior thyroid arteries through their laryngeal branches. These are accompanied by that system of nerves which controls the arterial supply to this locality for all purposes.

Among these effects we find thickenings and enlargements of the membrane and muscles, the result of blood being retained in this locality when it should have passed on and up to the brain. I reason that if there is no contraction of the muscles and ligaments connecting the neck with the head there will be no obstruction, provided the atlas and axis are in their normal position. I further reason that with the channels all open the blood will be carried to the inner chamber of the cranium, provided there is no interference from surgical injuries or tumefactions inside the cranium.

Prognosis.—The general history and statistics of laryngitis show it to be a very dangerous and fatal disease in a large percentage of cases, especially so in some of its forms. Such was my experience and observation for many years during which time I treated these laryngeal diseases as an allopath. But since I have reasoned about these diseases as a mechanic and treated them as a mechanic my success in handling them has been far more satisfactory. So far as my memory reaches and at least during the past thirty years I can say that when I have had an early opportunity to treat a child or a person suffering with laryngeal disease, and who enjoyed fairly good health otherwise, I have lost none of them.

Treatment.—I always begin my treatment in such diseases of the neck as loss of voice, sore throat or inflammation of the larynx by the most careful exploration of the eight upper dorsal vertebrae, their ribs, their articulation, their ligaments and their musculature, then travel up to the region of the clavicles. The first and second ribs on both sides I carefully explore and never stop until I know their articulation is perfectly correct with both spine and sternum. They must be normal. Here I halt and use all of my skill and intelligence to ascertain and know that the articulations of the clavicles are absolutely correct. The outer ends must not be too far back nor the sternal end dropped down inside against the neck. At this point I never rest until I know I have secured a perfect adjustment.

I pass on up the neck and know that the lower joint (or the seventh cervical) of the neck articulates perfectly with the first dorsal. It must be absolutely normal with no twist either backward or forward. Then I journey on up through the cervical region carefully searching for variations until I reach the axis and atlas and make sure their articulations are perfectly normal. Now I have arrived at a point in the exploration which will call for the most perfect knowledge of the true articulation of the atlas with the occiput. I have previously described what I look for and as you have all been thoroughly instructed in the adjustment of such variations as are possible in these conditions it is not necessary for me to go into detail, yet it may be as well if I specialize in some particulars.

Having the chin drawn forward and downward gently raise the hyoid bone up being careful to do no bruising or injuring of the parts. Draw the bone carefully forward, one side at a time, after having loosened the structures about it and under the inferior maxillary bone. When I wish to adjust these bones from any variation back to the normal I generally place one hand back of the patient's head letting the fingers come well around to the transverse processes then I gently lean the head towards my fingers, away from myself, holding my fingers firmly on the hard processes and giving the neck a very slight twisting motion backward and forward until I am satisfied that all ligaments are free and not held in any abnormal position. At this particular place in my treatment I place the fingers of one hand on the front side of the neck and the fingers of my other hand in behind and between the inferior maxilla and the atlas and axis, then gently but firmly pull hard enough to separate the head from the inferior maxillary tangle in which I generally find it. I nearly always find this locality under the ear in a very constricted condition.

Before I leave this subject I would draw your attention to the lower dorsal and the eleventh and twelfth ribs, the lumbar vertebrae and on down to the sacrum. Adjust and see that every articulation is normal and in order, with the view in mind that the kidneys can act with renovating freedom. All this work can be done without torturing or hurting your patient, and I want to say right here that the more you hurt the patient the less good you will accomplish. You must not hurt your patients while you are treating them. My observation has been that he who hurts his patient shows his lack of skill.

DISEASES OF THE PHARYNX.

Etiology.—In entering upon the important subject of diseases of the pharynx and accompanying organs and glands, I will give you one positive statement based upon a long experience. In my opinion the same cause—ligation—is parent of every one of the diseases which have been given you in detail.

When the arterial blood is detained in the thyroid system bulky growths appear. The arterial blood is the highest order of living fluid and should pass from the heart on to its destination and return without any obstruction whatever. It is a living substance whose function is to build or construct, and when hindered in its passage through the capillaries and into the veins it proceeds to build up abnormal growths and structures.

Should the venous system be obstructed congestion, inflammation, pus formation would be the result. This same law extends to the deep and superficial cervical glands, the tonsils, the auditory and nasal membranes. The blood must go and come without interference. The business of the osteopath is to know that the blood has an unobstructed flow through the arteries, capillaries and veins.

One etiological factor of disease of the pharynx is obstructed venous circulation, hindering the blood drainage from its structures back to the heart. This venous blood, as the student well knows, should not be tolerated to remain long enough for stagnation, fermentation and inflammation, because when it is detained by any sort of ligation, pressure or constriction, it loses its vitality and is in a condition that allows it to set up the process of decomposition. Thus we have the irritation caused by a venous congestion in the parts, which soon passes on to inflammation, fermentation, decomposition and sloughing of the pharyngeal membrane.

Prognosis.—The prognosis for relief in pharyngeal disease is good when the patient is early in the hands of an osteopath who understands the law and the function of the arterial and venous systems, and is mechanical enough to be able to adjust the structures to their normal condition. As to the length of time, I would say many patients are relieved in twenty-four hours, some in twelve. It is according to the length of time the patient has been affected, also to the recuperative power of the patient.

Examination.—On my examination, in cases of pharyngeal diseases, I find the atlas, the axis and sometimes the cervical vertebrae down as low as the fifth bulging forward toward the inferior maxilla. I find heavy contraction of the muscles of the atlas and axis. I find a depression of the back of the neck caused by the contracture of the recti and other muscles attached to the base of the skull. In proportion to the irritation and the extension of the contracture downward along the muscles do they push the cervical vertebrae forward. Then I look at the clavicles. I generally find the acromian and sternal ends drawn far back, particularly at the outer end at the scapula where it can be felt too far back on the acromian process, and sometimes I find it pulled clear back of the acromian producing heavy pressure on the venous system as it descends towards the heart. This pressure is generally strong enough to bring the venous blood to a halt in all parts of the neck and its structures clear up and into the brain.

Treatment.—In treating pharyngeal diseases, I first adjust the clavicles at both ends. I also adjust all of the ribs of each side from the first to the fifth. In adjusting the atlas and axis I place the fingers of one hand on their anterior processes and the fingers of my other hand I place behind the angle of the jaw and gently pull the jaw forward from the neck until I am sure there is no obstruction to the approach or the return of blood from the brain. If the fingers on the anterior processes hurt the patient, put one hand behind and under the back of the head and the other beneath the chin and pull the head forward. Then I see that the lower ribs from the eighth to the twelfth are all left in a normal condition. I am very careful to have a normal adjustment of the whole lumbar region.

Then I place my hand on the front of the abdomen in the region of the symphysis pubis where I make gentle pressure for a short time. Then I glide my hand upward along the course of the ureters to the region of the kidneys. I do this in order that I may take all irritation off of the ureters. As a general rule I do this once a day and in very, acute cases oftener. When my patient cools down and breaks out into a pleasant perspiration with the kidneys active, I think I have finished my work, but I keep close watch over the patient for several days on account of the changes in temperature which can occur in the house or in the weather.

In regard to diet, for the first few days give mild soups or gruels. When the throat is very sore and tender have a dish of sweet gruel handy so that the patient can take a swallow of it very often to allay the irritation that is caused by the raw surfaces touching each other. This treatment applies to all of the diseases of the pharynx in patients of all ages, if taken in time.

ACUTE TONSILLITIS.

Definition.—Cynanche tonsillaris; inflammation of the tonsil; quinsy.
—Dunglison.

Definition of Cynanche Tonsillaris.—Inflammatory sore throat, common quinsy; characteristic symptoms of this affection are swelling and florid redness of the mucous membrane of the fauces, and especially of the tonsils; painful and impeded deglutition, with inflammatory fever. It is generally ascribed to cold, and is a common affection of cold and temperate climates; it usually goes off by resolution, but frequently ends in suppuration. Ordinary tonsillitis is usually of no consequence, requiring merely rest and the observance of the antiphlogistic regimen; when more violent—in addition to this—local bleeding, purgatives, inhalation of the steam of medicated water, emollient gargles, and rubefacients externally or sinapisms or blisters are called for. When suppuration must inevitably occur an opening should be made into the abscess as soon as pus shall have formed. If the patient is being suffocated by the tumefaction, tracheotomy may be necessary.
—Dunglison.

Etiology.—The factors which tend to cause such an enlargement of the tonsils as is seen in acute tonsillitis are in my opinion the action of atmospheric changes, the result of which is a contraction of the neck muscles sufficient to draw the inferior maxilla too far backward. This interferes with the normal flow of blood to the head and so causes an overcharging of the arteries to the tonsils which is followed by congestion. The atmospheric shock affects the skin, then continues to the fascia affecting its nerve and blood supply. It then continues on to the muscles and their nerve and blood supply. This contraction holds the fluids shut up in the tissues till stagnation and decomposition set in.

Pathological Anatomy.—In some cases but one tonsil is affected and it is much swollen. When both are equally attacked the swelling may extend until the median line is reached and there is danger of suffocation. The tonsils are red, and show yellow patches on their surface. They are sensitive and in severe cases become quite painful. When suppuration occurs the tonsils soften, which shows that the venous blood has decomposed.

Prognosis—In acute tonsillitis the prognosis is favorable. Especially is it so when the osteopath has the case any where near its inception. Relapses are not so likely to occur under osteopathic treatment and permanent hypertrophy cannot result, provided the osteopath clears away all obstruction to-the normal supply of arterial blood and the perfect drainage of the venous blood.

Examination.—Commence at the lower jaw. See that it is in place and is not pressing backward upon the superior cervical ganglion and interfering with the vasomotor nerve supply to the tonsils. Examine the atlas. See that the occiput articulates perfectly with it. Take each cervical vertebra separately and test its integrity. Examine also the first four upper dorsal vertebrae and the ribs attached to them. Look well to the clavicles. See that their sternal ends are well thrown forward and in good articulation with the sternum. Then examine well the hyoid bone. See that no contractured muscle holds it out of its normal place permitting it to press upon nerves or blood vessels.

Treatment.—Let the osteopath's first work be to adjust the inferior maxillary bone, as previously described. Turn the head slightly to one side and draw the lower jaw well forward. See that the structures between it and the upper cervical vertebrae are set free on both sides of the neck in order that the flow of blood through the carotid artery on its way to the brain may pass on unobstructed and also secure a free passage of blood back through the jugular veins, draining thoroughly all structures.

Adjust whatever slight irregularity you find in the cervical and upper dorsal regions. Bring your clavicles well up and forward. Look carefully to your upper four ribs and see that they are perfectly adjusted on both sternum and spine. Free the hyoid bone from any contractured muscle which could bind it. Treat your patient once or twice a day in severe cases and when the case is a very obstinate one stick to it until you obtain good circulation. Then go to the lumbar region and treat there to open the excretories. See that the lumbar vertebrae are in line and that the floating ribs are well up and in their proper places. Do all your work in the neck region from the outside. Give these patients good plain nutritious food. I find the light gruels of much use. Have it so they can take occasional sips. Its action over the inflamed surface is to protect them from irritation.

CHRONIC TONSILLITIS.

Definition Chronic Catarrhal Tonsillitis.—A form attended by permanent hypertrophy, and usually requiring tonsillectomy.

—Dorland.

Etiology—Tonsillitis in its chronic form is a condition which is caused by the tonsils being kept from a normal arterial supply and a good venous drainage. Inasmuch as the arteries to the tonsils are supplied with vasomotor impulses through the superior cervical ganglion, it is plain to be seen that vascular disturbances would follow any lesion which would disturb the normal functioning of this ganglion.

Prognosis.—The prognosis of chronic tonsillitis is favorable in the hands of a skillful osteopath. The restoration of normal blood supply and perfect drainage to and from the organs lessens the liability to contract colds or to the recurrence of the acute form of the disease known as tonsillitis.

Treatment—Use very gentle, firm pressure with the flat of the fingers (not permitting the fingers to slide or slip on the skin) on the sides and in front of the neck, in order that the fluid channels both ways be opened up. Give this treatment every other day. Raise the clavicles. Attend to the upper ribs and all of the cervical vertebrae and secure perfect mechanical adjustment of all structures of the neck as well as of the thoracic region. See that the entire excretory system of the body is doing its proper work. Open up the ureters as you have been taught. Treat the splanchnic area thoroughly.

DEPOSITS IN THE TONSILS.

Etiology.—When deposits are formed in the tonsils, lesions of the atlas and axis are found. I have found the clavicles entirely off and back of the acromian processes. Generally the sternal end is pulled back against the structures of the neck and pressing so hard as to practically ligate all vessels whose function is to drain the tonsils and their surrounding structures. The outer end being off its proper articulation there is nothing to hinder the muscles from drawing the clavicles tight against the neck, which prohibits the return oi the fluids from the tonsils. It matters little to me what is deposited there. My object is to remove all obstructions to the circulation of the arterial, venous and lymphatic fluids.

Treatment.—Do not leave the clavicles in any abnormal condition at either end. Bring them well forward and off the neck. With hand flat on side of the neck, gentle pressure in the region of the tonsil will relieve any congestion or deposit found there. Adjust the first two ribs at their articulation with the transverse processes of the vertebrae. Carefully do this on both sides of the neck. The blood must have freedom and when that is secured it can be depended upon for repairs.

GOITER.

Definition.—Enlargement of the thyroid body, causing a swelling in the front part of the neck; bronchocele. The disease is endemic in Switzerland, the Alps of Savoy, in Styria, etc., being often accompanied by the condition known as cretinism.

—*Dorland.*

Definition.—A goiter, as I understand it, is an enlargement of the thyroid gland. It is an effect following the failure of the arterial blood to reach the brain and return normally.

Etiology.—Tumors and tumefaction of the neck with pressure on the trachea, esophagus, pneumogastric nerves, the jugular veins, the innominate veins and the axillary veins, arteries and nerves is the result of manubrium, clavicles, ribs or upper dorsal vertebrae having lost their normal position by violence. A strangulation of venous blood of the brain and neck follows such variations from normal articulations of the bones. They press upon all of the blood-vessels-that go through the neck to the brain and produce enlargement of the muscles and glands of the neck, head and face.

A goiter is no mystery to a mechanic. Protrusion of the eyes or strangulated breathing caused by such pressure ceases to be a mystery to the man who reasons as a mechanic. A goiter is a product and no mystery. You may say exophthalmic, soft, hard, fibrinous, but "what has produced it" is the question of the mechanic who seeks the cause and proves the correctness of his conclusion by the result, which is the obliteration of the tumors and normalizing of brain, lung and heart, all of which vouch for his ability as a mechanic.

An enlargement of the thyroid gland is due to a failure of the carotid arteries to deliver the blood inside the cranium. The blood must be normally delivered. No guess work or may-be-so's can be tolerated for one single minute or it will deposit an excess at some other place; then congestion will result and new growths will occur because of the building properties of the arterial blood.

A very common cause of goiter is the slipping of the first rib off, back and under the transverse process of the upper dorsal vertebrae. This allows the first rib to obstruct the drainage from the thyroid gland to the heart. If that venous blood stops in the glands they will soon get abnormally large, then we say goiter. Often we have the clavicles pulled back against the veins and nerves of the neck and esophagus, then we have exophthalmic goiter; and so on through the list of diseases of the thyroid gland.

Prognosis.—In the majority of cases osteopathic treatment of goiter has shown marked success. Disappearance of the glandular enlargement has sometimes followed the first treatment. The osteopath is to promise nothing more than to do the best he or she can with any and all kinds of goiters. The results of my work in this line have been very satisfactory. By the process here given to you I have removed many. You will find many goiters which have been medicated by outward and inward applications and by the use of the syringe until they have become very hard. In such cases the prognosis is less favorable. Should you find a very hard stony substance in the center of the gland you have a surgical case.

Examination.—In examining your goiter patient you are to carefully examine all the structures of the neck. See that the cranium sets in its normal position on the atlas; that all the cervical vertebrae are in normal articulation; so also the first four dorsal vertebrae and their connections with the ribs; and the ribs in their articulation with the sternum. Look well to your clavicles and scapulae. Attend to the lower maxillary bone; see that it articulates as it should. Examine the masseter and buccinator muscles; see that they are not in a contractured state and pulling the jawbone backward causing it to press upon the blood vessels and obstructing them in their work.

Treatment.—The best way to reduce the size of a goiter is to get out of it the blood, water and other fluids which are being held there by ligation. What is a ligation? Answer: anything which by weight, pressure or strain stops the flow of blood when it is running from the thyroid gland back to the heart. In treating your patient who has simple goiter, adjust the inferior maxilla. See that it is not pressing on the ascending carotid artery. When you find that it is, adjust it by placing one hand behind the angle of the jaw the other on the chin. Ask the patient to open the mouth then push the chin down, the angle up and forward, with a slight twisting movement crossways, and be sure that the jaw is in its normal position. Be sure that the masseter and buccinator muscles are truly normal. Wrap a handkerchief around your thumb, place it inside the mouth on top of the teeth and gently press down, giving a slight rotary motion right and left.

Now as you have articulated the lower maxilla and it has regained its normal position you are ready to treat the atlas should it be found necessary; also the cervical vertebrae. You are to be very careful with your work here because the lower cervical vertebrae are often found pushed back so far that their spinous processes are even with those of the first dorsal. Seat your patient. Stand in front, having the patient's forehead against your breast, your hands at the back of the neck, fingers on the transverse processes of the cervical vertebrae. Then gently and carefully press the neck downward until you have that part well adjusted. Then you have the vertebral artery set at liberty. Now carefully adjust the sternal end of your clavicles and know for a certainty that they are not too far back or forward, nor out of place in any way and that they are not lying against any of the ascending or descending blood vessels. Now go to the outer ends of your clavicles and ascertain if they are in their proper places. See that they articulate with the acromian processes as they should and are not stopped behind the coracoid processes. Place one hand on the scapula, elevate the arm, bring it back say six inches above a horizontal position when the patient sits erect and then bring the arm with an upward tendency square toward the forehead. Or, stand your patient against a door jamb with his face toward you: Put your hand on his shoulder, push the arm back sufficient to make a gap or opening between the outer end of the clavicle and scapula and then bring the arm with an upward tendency square toward the forehead.

Now carefully examine to see if the first or second rib or both have not been pushed back, off and under their articular processes. Perfect articulation must be secured in all this part of the body or you are likely to fail to reduce the goiter. If a first rib falls under the transverse process, changes its position on the sternum and drops across an important draining blood vessel, you must have for your object the return of that rib to its normal place at both ends. If the spinal end is too far back, pull it forward; if the sternal end has fallen inside the sternum get it out. Be careful and know that there is no pressure from rib or clavicle on the draining vein.

Now back to the goiter itself. You must ever remember that you must not bruise the gland. Place your hand underneath the enlargement and very gently raise up with a slight squeezing movement. You will find the tissue has been shoved down towards the sternum by the weight of the glands. Get under those thin fibrous ligaments by gently drawing them up from the esophagus. Place your fingers so they will pass over, back and under the glands and give a gentle squeezing movement so the fluids will start to pass down and out of the glands. In case you have a soft goiter this gentle raising releases the contained fluid and you can expect a reduction in size. When I find goiters which contain concretions or stones it is my custom to simply adjust the bones of the neck and clavicles and stop there, letting the blood do what it will. As a result, much of the suffocation and difficulty in breathing is relieved, also some reduction in bulk.

EXOPHTHALMIC GOITER.

Definition.—Basedow's disease, Graves's disease, Bigbie's disease, Stokes's disease, Parkinson's disease, Marsh's disease, Parry's disease, anaemic protrusion of the eyeballs, cardiothyroid or anaemic exophthalmia. An anaemic condition, accompanied by protrusion of the eyeballs, palpitation of the heart and arteries, and tumefacation of the thyroid gland; is more frequent among women than men. It was, named by Trousseau, of Paris, after Dr. Graves, who first described it in 1835. Its etiology is still obscure; the disease is regarded as a sympathetic neurosis, possibly due to hypersecretion of the thyroid gland.

—Dunglison.

Etiology.—I will say to the osteopath that if he is any wiser after having read the theories of the medical authors on the subject of exophthalmic goiter he has succeeded in gaining Something where I have failed. The theories begin in supposition and continue in that strain without having made a single point with which a philosopher could conscientiously agree. The causes given as producing such effects are wholly untrustworthy from start to finish.

I am not satisfied to give an osteopathic doctor any advice in regard to exophthalmic goiter until I have given him something that sounds or looks as though I had explored the mechanical superstructure through which the blood is conducted from the heart to the gland, the brain, the eye, and distributed according to the needs of each organ. As the condition of the eye enters into the subject of our discussion, I will say or grant that the arterial supply to the brain is normal. If that be so why should the eye become congested or pushed out of its normal place or changed in appearance?

We know the normal head, neck and glands receive their blood supply through the ascending arterial system. We will have to hunt until we find a cause for this over-accumulation of fluid (or end enlargement of the glands) which by all methods of reasoning we find is an effect produced by the failure of the venous system to receive and carry the venous blood back to the heart. Every obstruction must be sought, discovered and removed or we will fail to give relief by reduction. To me this position is an undebatable one. I have been guided by this philosophy and have successfully treated exophthalmic goiter.

I have proven to my own mind that the venous system by not returning the blood is responsible for all the effects of this condition.

Prognosis.—The favorable results that I have obtained in my treatment of exophthalmic goiter under this philosophy (which is treating it as a mechanic or engineer would treat a machine which has from any cause become strained or obstructed in its ability to run to the rule of perfect mechanical harmony), have been very gratifying. Remember this, I am not talking to the engineer of the human body, giving him the benefit of the result of my labors. The probability of a cure is good in proportion to your ability as an operator to know the abnormal and to adjust this part of the human body to the truly normal.

Examination.—In the examination of an exophthalmic patient there is one question that should be always before the mind's eye of the operator, viz: What is the cause of this venous obstruction? The first thing that I would examine would be the sternal end of the clavicles. Know for a certainty that they are not thrown inside of the manubrium and therefore pressing upon the jugular, the thyroid or any other vein whose function is the drainage of fluid from the structures in question.

From the sternum I would go to-the acromian processes at the outer end of the clavicles and know for a certainty that they are not thrown off and back and held out of position by the coracoid process or any ligament or muscle. Examine with the greatest care the upper ribs, especially the first two, and never leave them until you know positively that they have been adjusted and are normally articulated at both ends.

Look for bony pressure on both the ascending arteries and descending veins. Examine the bony structure of the entire upper dorsal and cervical regions; the cranium as it articulates with the atlas; the inferior maxilla and the hyoid bone. Test the integrity of all of the musculature of the neck and see that it is free from contractures.

Treatment.—To successfully treat and give relief in the condition known as exophthalmic goiter I begin at the sternal end of the clavicles and make sure and know that their articulation with the sternum is absolutely correct. Should the sternal end be found pressing against any of the structures of the neck, pull it forward and out until its articulation is normal. If you consider there is no variation from normal then pass to the outer end of the clavicles and adjust their articulations with the acromian processes by the methods which I have given you. Or place your patient on his back on the treating table. Let an assistant hold firmly down to the table the shoulder opposite to the one being treated. Bring the arm up a little above the level of a line drawn across the breast from one shoulder to the other and bring the abnormal side on a strain by pushing the arm back towards the spine while the patient lies in this position. This will carry backward the scapulae and pull the one far enough from the outer end of the clavicle to make it fairly easy work to push it back into its articulation with the acromian process.

Patients suffering with exophthalmic goiter often show the sternum in a twisted condition. This condition you are to correct. Now by adjusting both ends of the clavicles and the manubrium you have taken off the pressure from the ascending carotid arteries which pressure no doubt often produces an enlargement of the aorta. In making this adjustment we have liberated the aorta and released a condition that would cause a strain on the heart. Remember that you are hereby relieving the carotid and thyroid arteries from oppressive disturbances.

Now we are ready to attend to the cervical region. Be careful to adjust any and every variation from the truly normal articulation of the first and second ribs in order that the vertebral arteries may receive and convey blood to its destination. Carefully adjust spine and ribs as far as the eighth dorsal. Be sure that there is a perfectly normal articulation of the facets of both sides. Now travel up the neck to the fifth cervical. Carefully adjust that because the nerves passing out from the spine in this location have much to do with the healthy condition of the eye.

Pass on up to the axis and atlas and make certain that the atlas is not shoved forward and off its articulation with the cranium producing ligation of the venous vessels which should drain the structures of the neck and head. Now treat the goiter by placing the flat of your hand (using the cushions of your fingers, not the tips), at the under side of the gland and gently draw the goiter up just far enough to allow blood and other substances to pass down from it. Gently press the enlarged gland and hold it in this position for a few moments using a very slight friction movement up and down the neck. As far as my experience or observation has led me there is no cause for variation from the normal in the heart action when the arterial system is absolutely free.

THYROIDITIS.

Definition.—Inflammation of the thyroid gland. —*Dunglison*.

Etiology.—In considering the cause of the condition known as thyroiditis I wish to dwell on the effects which follow when ribs, sternum or clavicles are thrown from their normal position by any cause, mechanical, postural, hard coughing, lifting or otherwise. Here is a condition which any philosopher would accept as a cause for a retention of blood or other fluids in the thyroid gland as well as in other glands of the neck, face and jaw. The congestion results in inflammation, fermentation and so on, known in this instance as thyroiditis.

The fact is we have the blood driven from the heart to the thyroid glands; the arterial doing the work of construction, while the venous blood is hindered and retained. We have as a result the bulky condition which would lead the operator directly to the clavicle, the manubrium, the scapula and to the first and second ribs. In every case of congestion of the thyroid gland he will find some of these at variance from the truly normal. The nerves and the lymphatic vessels must be just as free as the blood vessels in order to carry out their necessary and perfect work.

Prognosis.—Under proper treatment when a thorough drainage of the venous system of all the structures of the neck and head and especially of the thyroid gland is secured, all inflammation rapidly subsides. Your prognosis is favorable in all cases except such as have waited until the tissue changes have gone beyond redemption, and even then you can give relief.

Treatment.—The osteopathic treatment for thyroiditis is to attend to and adjust any and every structure muscle, bone or ligament which could in any manner, by pressure or otherwise, maintain an obstruction to the venous system, which should drain normally and perfectly the blood and lymph from the thyroid gland into the internal jugular and innominate veins, on to the superior vena cava and right auricle of the heart.

You are to make sure that the vessels from the gland back to the heart are unobstructed and able to carry out their normal function of drainage without which you cannot expect to get an abeyance of the inflammation. Perfect drainage and perfect arterial supply to nourish the structures are an absolute necessity in order to secure anything like a normal condition.

MYXEDEMA.

Definition.—A trophoneurotic condition characterized by general dropsy-like swelling, especially of the face and hands, caused by the presence of mucous fluid in the subcutaneous tissues. The swelling is hard and puffy and does not pit on pressure. The disease is associated with atrophy of the thyroid gland, and is apparently due to excess of mucin in the system. It is marked by dullness of mental faculties, sluggishness of movement, unsteadiness of gait, and thick speech.

—Dorland.

Etiology.—To find the causes which produce the effect called myxedema, or sporadic cretinism, search for the cut-off in the thyroid arteries whose business it is to supply nutrition to the gland itself. When arteries supply blood, and veins refuse to carry off drainage then we have fermentation, sore tonsils, congestion of the cervical glands generally, with a face puffed up by stagnation due to such a stoppage of the return fluids. Hence we have a long list of effects, which should all be under the head of strangulated circulation of blood in the neck, face, brain and all organs pertaining to the head. Put these effects all together and to me they are each and all the result of pressure on some artery or vein. This is my opinion of the cause which has produced this long list of effects.

In my opinion heredity has nothing to do with this condition except in so far as some people are born with slender bones, which are easily moved from their normal position, producing interference and obstruction to the perfect circulation. As to the falling off of the hair, I have long since told you that stagnation of blood in the venous system of the scalp is the cause of hair falling off and out.

Prognosis.—I will answer the question, is myxedema curable, by saying that from my observation and practice, I have gotten good results, clear skin, and a general improvement following the adjustment of the bones of the head, neck and upper chest, when they were kept in position any reasonable length of time. You must make some allowance for advanced age and also for any surgical injury which may have been done and is acting as a cause. In the cases which have come under my care I have hoped for and obtained good results. When you do your duty as a mechanic you will be pleased with the results of your efforts in myxedema, especially when you get the case in its early stages.

Examination.—Make an examination of your myxedematous patients for anything which could obstruct the carotid, thyroid or subclavian arteries. See that the musculature of the neck is free from contractions; that the cervical vertebrae are all normal; the upper dorsal and their ribs and the clavicles well articulated and that there is nothing to interfere with the normal flow of blood from the heart through the neck into the cranium and the return to the heart through the veins (especially the jugulars and their branches).

Treatment.—In the treatment already outlined for the glandular abnormalities of the neck, I have tried to emphasize that when you have a normal neck with an unobstructed flow of blood from the heart to the brain and all its organs, and there is no obstruction to the venous system by pressure at any point between the head and heart, your work is done.

I have told you as carefully as I know how that the clavicle and its articulations must be normal. The upper ribs must also be normal and from the atlas as low down as the fourth dorsal, or even lower, the articulations must be absolutely normal if you wish good results. We must reason as architects, act as mechanics, work as builders and engineers, and the results will be satisfactory in proportion to the thoroughness of our work. I have long since found in my treatment of such diseases as this one under consideration that nature is trustworthy in all its work.

THORACICS REGION

CLAVICLE ADJUSTMENTS.

To adjust the clavicle on either side, I lay my patient on his back on the treating table, or some solid substance. When the patient is not able to get onto the treating table, I generally place a book or something solid between the scapulae and the bed, simply to hold the scapulae solid. Then with the hollows of my hands placed on the front and upper part of the patient's shoulders, I bring down steady firm pressure which spreads them apart. After springing them, then with my left or right hand, according to the side I am on, I hook my fingers over the top or back of the convex surface of the clavicle. I am now in front of the patient and on the left side. It is an easy matter in this position to adjust, by placing the left hand on and behind the patient's left clavicle which is to be pulled forward, at the same time swing the patient's left arm outward. I take the patient's left arm in my right hand with my left fingers on the clavicle; then press the arm outward, holding my left fingers solid in the place just named. Now I bring the arm in line from the shoulder towards the face and head, swinging the arm on a circle over the head, and on back to a right angle with the body, push up tolerably strong and bring the arm back to the chin and your work is done.

I will give you another method. While the patient is lying on his back on the table draw the patient towards you far enough to bring the arm and shoulder on a line and a little off the table. Have an assistant bear down on opposite shoulder, and keep the body firmly on the table. You now have your patient in a position so that you can easily adjust the outer end of the clavicle. Bring the arm out from the body, place your fingers at the outer third of the clavicle, pull it toward you, and take the arm square back and toward the head of the table, gently but firmly. Be sure that the scapulae are bearing heavily on the table. You will find that carrying the arm backward will draw the clavicle out from the sternum; it will also draw the scapulae away from the acromian end of the clavicle. You can also do this while you have the arm at right angles and in a straight line from the body by bringing it down slowly and gently towards the floor; or use your thigh as a fulcrum in the axilla, bringing the arm across it as a lever. As you have separated the outer end of the clavicle from the acromian process which you should do in all dislocations of the outer end of the clavicle either above or below its, articulation with the scapula, hold your hand firmly on the clavicle and bring the arm up to the breast, on over the face, and up to the head. By this process I have no difficulty in adjusting the clavicles at both ends.

When you find surgical injuries at the acromian end of either of the clavicles or scapulae you must work with great caution in order not to set up an inflammation in this region. This process will generally correct the clavicle to the condition of normal articulation. By this method I adjust the scapula and what is known as "winged scapula" disappears. The cause of "winged scapula" is partial or complete dislocation of the outer end of the clavicle which is intended to hold the scapula in its normal position. Thus we have a scapula, the clavicle and the sternum adjusted. By this same process the long head of the biceps and other muscles that are sometimes the seat of rheumatic or other soreness are adjusted and the soreness disappears.

An adjustment by this process takes off all pressure of the clavicles on the front side of the neck, and frees up the circulation, and is very important to know when you are dealing with asthma, goiter, glandular swelling, loss of voice, irritable cough and other troubles of the neck. Particularly is this effective and necessary if you wish to reduce obesity.

My choice of clavicle adjustments is to treat the clavicle while the patient is in an erect position. It is one I often use when I have an acromian dislocation with the outer end of the clavicle far back on the acromian process.

I stand my patient in the open doorway, with his back against the flat surface of the door-jamb. While in this position I have an assistant press firmly against the opposite shoulder from the one which I wish to adjust. Then, grasping the arm at the elbow I bring it forward, upward and outward, keeping my fingers as before described on and back of the outer third of the clavicle. I draw the clavicle forward while taking the arm strongly up and out, and when I know that the scapula is pushed far enough to make a separation between it and the acromian end of the clavicle I bring the arm backward and downward to the side holding the fingers on the clavicle as described. Then I push up on the arm with sufficient force to bring the scapula up above the acromian end of the clavicle. While in this position, I bring the arm across the face with an upward motion. Now let the arm fall at the side and the work is done.

When the clavicular dislocation is of long standing such a manipulation should be given once or twice each week in order to loosen up the muscles and ligaments enough to replace the clavicle to its normal position. I have here given you a rough statement in plain language, and would advise you to practice on normal cases in order that you may be familiar with the movements just described. There may be other methods just as good.

This method of adjusting both ends of the clavicle is my choice of all in my long experience in doing this work. The more normal shoulders you manipulate and experiment with, the less confusion and embarrassment you will have with abnormal cases. Right here I want to emphasize that you must not use awkward movements or violence or hurt your patient. Such procedure will cause your patient to be disgusted, not only with you, but with osteopathy, and you will lose your patient. Once for all I want to say that you do not need to hurt or torture any patient when adjusting a bone or any part of the body.

LECTURE ON THE LUNGS.

Definition of Lung.—Essential organ of respiration which is double and occupies the two sides of the chest. The lungs, which are of a spongy, soft, flexible, compressible, and dilatable structure, fill exactly the two cavities of the thorax, and are separated from each other by the mediastinum and the heart. The right lung, which is shorter and broader than the left, is divided by two oblique fissures into three unequal lobes, lobi or alae pulmonum. The left has only two lobes, and consequently only one fissure. At the internal surface of these organs, which is slightly concave, there is about the middle a pedicle formed by the bronchia and the pulmonary vessels, and called by anatomists the root of the lungs. Essentially, the lungs are composed of prolongations and ramifications of the bronchia and of the pulmonary arteries and veins, the divisions of which are supported by a fine areolar tissue.

When the surface of the lungs is examined in a clear light, we may see, even through the pleura, that their parenchyma is formed by the aggregation of a multitude of small vesicles, of an irregularly spheroid or ovoid shape, full of air, and separated by white and opaque septa, constituting lozenge-shaped spaces, which are called lobules—lobuli or insulae pulmonales—and which are separated by interlobular areolar tissue. These lobules do not communicate with each other. The series of air-sacs connected with the extremity of each bronchial twig has been called a lobulette. The vesicles are called air-cells, air-vesicles or lung-vesicles, spiramenta or spiramina, or cellulae pulmonum. They who regard the bronchial tubes as terminating in elongated cavities have termed those cavities air-sacs, infundibula, Malpighian vesicles, terminal cavities, etc., and the cup-like cavities observed in these have been called alveoli. They are the air-cells.

Along the partitions or septa is deposited in greater or less quantity black pulmonary matter, as it has been called, which seems to be normal. Sometimes it is seen in points, at other times in spots. The color of the lungs varies according to age and other circumstances. In youth it is more red, and afterwards grayish or bluish, often as if marbled. The pleura pulmonalis is their investing membrane. The air is carried to the lungs by means of the trachea and bronchi. The black, venous blood which requires oxygenation is conveyed to the lungs from the heart by the pulmonary artery, and when it has undergone this change it is returned to the heart by the pulmonary veins. The blood-vessels inservient to the nutrition of the lungs are the bronchial arteries. The pulmonary lymphatics are very numerous. Some are superficial, others deep-seated. They pass for the most part into the bronchial ganglions or glands. Nerves are furnished by the pulmonary plexus. The lungs are respiratory organs in which venous blood is oxygenated.

—Dunglison.

Fundamentals of truth are only obtained by studious attention to business. Thus the mind grows in the art of arranging the facts in such order that one truth after another falls in line until doubt gives place to knowledge. Then we are able to demonstrate that our conclusion is no longer debatable, and doubt and hope give place to the newborn truth. The man who succeeds does more than follow a theory. His motto is "demonstration or nothing". If we do not know how or why the lungs act, we do know that when the lung or heart fails man dies. The whole lung system, how it acts and what it does by its action has been one of the unsolved mysteries in the history of man. Man has surely reasoned that a lung is a part of a machine, the heart another, and it is equally true of all other organs. No part, great or small, in the whole machine can be taken away and perfect functioning follow in life's action. If we expect perfect health we must look for any variation and keep all parts in condition to do the work they can do when in line. I am not writing to tell the reader what the lung is by quoting what authors have said on the lung and its diseases, because with all this recorded wisdom, the people die just as fast today as at any time. I will state my opinion even if it is not yours nor theirs. I want to feel the branding-iron of reason, then I will know the truth by the depth of the burn

The lung, to me, is a most important organ. I have cut loose for a time to ask all philosophers and Nature to unbosom a few of the secrets of the lung. We all know a great many elementary facts pertaining to the lungs, where they are situated, their size and form, that they draw air into them and that they push it out. At this point the needle of our compass trembles and centers on nothing. We know that in good health the lungs act in an undisturbed manner. Where this is the condition and the heart and other organs and parts of the body are undisturbed, we are bold to say that we have and enjoy good health. We know we can look upon the lung as one of the organs, beings, or personalities of life. We know that immediately following a wound from a bullet, a knife or any other force that would produce a surgical injury, health suffers in proportion to the extent of the injury. Other injuries are just as dangerous as the surgical, such as inhaling deadly gases or being filled by water, blood or any other substance. The result is death, instantaneous or progressive. Then come in the natural processes such as a strong and normal arterial supply with a venous return which fails to carry away substances that should be passed off. We know the result is to accumulate bodies which require space in proportion to the size of the substance retained. Then atmospheric changes, eruptive fevers and many other causes produce retention, stagnation, inflammation, fermentation and a deposit of such substances as are left at the end of fermentation.

I have taken up the human lung to investigate and treat it as though it were a part of the machinery of life. I have traveled on this road for many years. At first I was very much disappointed to find that when I properly adjusted the spine with the ribs misery disappeared and my patient with pleurisy or pneumonia got well without a drop or a dose of any drug; I was surprised, disappointed, and glad, to know I had discovered that when all bones were in place and joints perfectly articulated, the whole body was a machine and could manufacture and apply all substances necessary to keep it in repair and health. One would say "what did you look for?" I explored spine and ribs to ascertain if any variations could be found. I never failed to find the variation that was the cause of pneumonia or inflammation of either side of the lungs. I also discovered that in such atmospheric changes as produced cold, pleuro-pneumonia, croup, scarlet fever and so oh, some one or many of the ribs on the suffering side were off from their proper place of articulation. Also in a very great majority of the cases of pleuro-pneumonia these variations were confined to the right side, lung and pleura. It matters not to the operator on which side the misery is located; until he finds and corrects all ribs and vertebrae on that side, he will fail. He is not likely to fail to give relief if he knows his business and proceeds accordingly. Otherwise he will resort to drugs, acknowledge his incompetency, disgust his patients and friends with that which he claimed to understand while his work proved the contrary.

An osteopath should always remember that his highest attainment is that of the well informed machinist and he should always feel that he is the judge who presides over the court of inquiry. This court is convened for the purpose of inspection of some part of the very wisely constructed machine whose parts, in order to do absolutely perfect functioning, must and shall be normal in form and place. Now I will say that so far as the human body is concerned, he is a well qualified master mechanic, who knows the difference between perfection and imperfection, both in the structure and functioning of the whole body, all its organs, separate and combined.

By way of the catechising instructor let me ask you before you take the responsibility to examine, diagnose and treat any case, to answer me a few questions. First classify and separately inquire of yourself what is expected of each organ in the functioning of life. What is the brain? Where is it? What is its use? Where is the spinal cord located? How long is it? Where does it begin? Where does it end? How many branches does it throw off from the occiput to the coccyx? What nerves could you injure by pressure, by bruising or any other ordinary injury? What nerve would cut off vision; cut off motion of the tongue; the power to swallow; the power of speech; the power to breathe; the power to move an arm; to move the head to the right or to the left or any other direction? If you know this, you know what impediment to look for. If not, you have no opinion until you shall have consulted your anatomy and physiology and refreshed your mind on the location and destination of every blood-vessel and every nerve on which the parts just mentioned depend. Then you can wisely proceed; give your opinion, your diagnosis, do your work and get the results hoped for.

Now let me ask you some other questions: What is your throat for? What is, its use? What is the windpipe for, and its use? What is the stomach for? Of what use are the bowels, both great and small? Of what use is the liver? What is its blood supply? What does it do? What do you expect of it? What is the spleen for? What benefit is it to the pancreas for normal life? Where does it get its supply to send back life? Of what use are the kidneys? If they are the batteries to drain off the impure waters, where are their nerve and blood supply? Where would you expect to shut off the nerve and blood supply to either or both of them? Of what use is the omentum? Of what use is the peritoneum? Where does it get its blood supply? How is that blood returned?

Suppose the supply is good and the return bad, could you expect good results and good work in the abdomen? Say no, and go on.

Now let me draw your attention to that organ called the lung. I want you to give attention to the question that I propose to ask you as an operator. When food has been received in the mouth, passed to the stomach and through all the vital processes of digestion and separation, and has been collected as chyle in the receptaculum chyli, delivered to the heart, mixed and passed on to the lungs, don't you see that their great work is to purify this chyle? We find the substances taken up and conducted to the heart by way of the thoracic duct. That substance is not pure enough to become arterial blood out of which all the parts of the animal economy are kept in form and force. Stop and think for just a moment that the fiat coming from the great Architect of the universe says this in thunder tones to the mind of the philosopher, "Perfection is expected, must and shall be shown in every atom of arterial blood."

Remember this, friendly operator, that when this blood leaves the lung it lives and acts as atoms or seeds of life. It has that quality or it could not prove it by its works. Thus the importance of perfect adjustment of every rib, and every vertebra from the head to the coccyx, or the work will fail to show perfection in place, form and function in some part of the body. Thus you see that failure of the lung to produce and the heart to send forth pure arterial blood is a cause of tracheal diseases, throat diseases, lung diseases, heart diseases, diseases of any organ or of the whole abdomen. Pure arterial blood is to me nothing more nor less than the living seeds of life, as much so as the seed of the mustard, wheat or any vegetable seed known to the agriculturist. You must have good seed or bad crops. Thus the lung, the garden spot of seed production, must be absolutely correct and the abdomen from which all substances are obtained by this lung must be in normal condition or the lung has poor material from which to make arterial blood on whose shoulders all animated nature leans for its existence. I am not giving this advice to tell you where to punch, pull or rub. This is to prepare you to become an explorer and a judge of first the normal then the abnormal. When you comprehend this you will know of your own ability what moves to make and what results to expect.

THE ACTION OF THE LUNGS.

(A lecture delivered to the dissecting class.)

After having demonstrated some of the actions of the lungs to a large number of students who are qualified because they have just closed a thorough and well directed course in dissection of the human body for this purpose, made acquainted by knife and observation with all the organs, divisions and functions of the body, I feel that they are among our most competent jurors to decide upon the philosophy of the action of the lungs as I understand it and have tried to explain as best I could. I have spoken of the probable power of the one lung to act for a time independent of the other, which is undoubtedly inactive during the chemical action of the substances in the lung just indicated. Now I will speak of the voluntary and involuntary powers of the lungs which will be seen and better comprehended by a careful review of the two pneumogastric nerves, each nerve being wholly independent of the other, the left nerve going to the left lung and the right going to the right lung, which completes the preparation for united or separate action of the lungs.

I think during conversation both lungs can be brought into service at the will of the speaker or singer, and in general conversation I am fully satisfied that when we desire, the full power of both lungs gets into action; the chemical substances in the lungs uniting with the atmospheric air on inspiration produces explosion, the result of chemical action converting into gas those substances contained in the lungs that are of no further use in sustaining life. I think that the combustion produces a gas that is used for vocal purposes and a great deal more in bulk than is taken into the lung as common atmosphere. Thus a short breath of atmospheric air keeps up this continual explosion and generates the gas by which long conversations are kept up. I think at will we can bring into action both lungs and generate gas for conversational purposes. Also, I think that during sleep one lung can and does alternate and act independent of the other for a time, receives atmospheric air and throws off the impurities that should be cast out from the lungs and receives fresh air. After the absorbents have taken up the purified substances necessary to

92

healthy blood and ejected the impure, and filled the lungs, then the other lung inhales the atmospheric air which unites with the substances in the lung and separates the impure from the good and throws off what we call foul breath, and refills with pure air to continue the process as above described.

When I commenced to reason and treat on this line, I felt it would be a journey traveled for many miles without company, because no pen so far as I know has ever traveled over the road that I am trying to blaze out to the understanding of the student, who though he be fine in anatomy, fine in physiology, yet is only a beginner when his attention is drawn to the peculiar condition of the lung or lungs. No one has ever told me that one lung can act while the other is silent. No one has ever told me that both could act at once. No author has ever been able to tell me what the real function of the lung is, but as I have raised the lone star often since I found and explored Nature's law by osteopathy, I have no hesitancy in running this star up, because I believe it to be one of the most brilliant of all constellations to be explored by the telescope of reason. Much of it is yet new to me, and I expect that it will grow brighter until it will be one of the day stars of light and life in lung diseases.

I have seen enough truth by my feeble method of investigation to know that we are in the presence of one of the most sublime truths ever beheld by the eye of man. I hope that in the future when combating diseases of the lungs we will be more successful. I am compelled to say that all pathologists, all physiologists, all writers on lung diseases, their causes and their cures, to me have been unsatisfactory and unreliable in results, because when I followed the tenets and practice of the same, I found I was with all the rest—in a humiliating defeat. Since I began to treat the lung as a machine I have had results far beyond anything I could hope for. In the treatment of asthma, pneumonia, croup, diphtheria, pleurisy and through the whole list of lung diseases, I find that Nature is a trust worthy leader, and there is much hope even for the consumptive.

I will say in conclusion to this class, that the day is not far off when the osteopath who is consulted by a consumptive, can tell him, "Yes, I can relieve you for the reason that I know the cause of your trouble." Students, I think we have discovered the key to the mystery.

LECTURE ON THE LUNGS.

(Delivered to dissecting class.)

Gentlemen and ladies of this class, your knives have laid open for your inspection every atom of flesh in every organ and part of man's body from skin to the bone. You have traced all muscles from origin to insertion. You know the nerve and blood supply of all of them. Also your scalpels have opened all organs of the body and with your microscope your eyes have seen all forms. By your physiology you have learned much of the functioning of each organ separately and combined, but much is yet to be learned before we know just how each organ performs its work. Right here we will draw your attention to the lungs and ask a few questions whose answers you will not find in any work on anatomy, physiology, pathology nor philosophy to this date, or at least I have failed to find them.

Questions.—When we breathe do we fill all five of the lobes of the lungs with atmospheric air at once, and how may we know if this is so? Why is it that in pneumonia the right lung is more often the first attacked? Why is it in a post-mortem examination of tuberculosis we find the left lung the seat of attack and showing so many tubercular deposits? Does the atmospheric air fill more than the three lobes of the right lung when we breathe and take in air at a very low temperature, say thirty to forty degrees below zero? Does it look reasonable to you that both lobes of the left lung lying right against the heart would be filled with air at the temperature indicated? Do you think the left lung could take in atmosphere at such a temperature and not shock the nerves of the heart? Let us ask the question as a mechanic, why are the two lobes of the left lung so much smaller than the three lobes of the right? Is this a provision of Nature to not shock the nervous system of the heart with too great a quantity of cold atmospheric air? The mechanical philosopher would say yes. We all know that the left lung is in a much warmer place than the right; therefore, we believe this is an important provision of Nature for warming less than two-fifths of the air inhaled. Doesn't it look very reasonable to you that the lobes of the right lung receive and warm the air of low temperature, and that pneumonia is the effect of chilled of frost bitten lungs on the right side?

Is it not reasonable to think that the left lung is not so sensitive as the right lung and is the separator of impure deposits that come with the blood that supplies the two lobes of that side? Is it not reasonable to suppose that the left lung being smaller and having less vital energy allows chyle and other substances to be retained, fermented, separated, and so form tubercles from the cheesy matter that is contained in the fluid substances? Will some philosopher tell us how many cubic inches of air comes out when we inhale two hundred at each breath? Does combustion of substances while in the lung generate gas? If not, how does the talker speak so long and loud with one breath? How many cubic inches of air or gas will one cubic inch of powder produce? How many barrels of steam will one barrel of water make at twelve hundred degrees of heat? Do we inspire one half of the wind we use when we talk? Is the lung a generator of gas in addition to its other powers? When the lung fails to generate gas by combustion of waste matter that comes to it will deposits follow and tubercles appear? If this be true we have some clew toward solving the question what is consumption? Answer: the lack of combustion.

It is very reasonable when we look at the form of the lungs and their size, all encased in pleural sacs to find those pleural sacs strong, elastic and well supplied with arteries and nerves. We then reason that those sacs can and do dilate and contract to suit the action of the lungs inhaling and exhaling. Only one question with an affirmative answer is required to establish one of the greatest truths found in Nature which will prove that she never fails to prepare for all demands in animal life. This being true we have a well grounded hope for the reduction of the ravages and mortality caused by consumption. Do both steam chests of an engine blow off at the same time? Do both piston heads of a locomotive move in the same direction at the same time? Or does the entering steam at one end push the piston head back, forcing the steam out of the other end of the cylinder? If so, why not reason that the two lungs represent a steam chest of a stationary engine? You know that the entering steam presses the exhausted steam out at the exhaust or wind pipe. Why not expect the lungs to do likewise when the law is the same in both cases? To keep our lungs or steam chests in motion by keeping all parts in place is the work of the skillful engineer, or osteopath, in all diseases of the head, neck, chest, abdomen and limbs.

In connection with this subject and with the philosophy of the lungs, the three lobes of the right side and two of the left, I wish to emphasize that my observation for a great number of years, and in particular the last twenty-five years, has convinced me that the prevailing system and practice of medicine has been far worse than a failure in diseases of the lungs; which embraces every degree of soreness in the trachea, lobes, gland, nerve and blood supply of the lungs, throat and neck. It matters not what we call it, tonsillitis, diphtheria, croup, catarrh or any other term, the results as to the remedies are unsatisfactory and I think always will be until we change our tactics. I have seen and felt this to be the true condition if we depended upon any drug, diet, change of climate or any other means or method such as washes, gargles, drinks and so on.

I am satisfied that we have traveled far enough without a compass and have been willing to confide in and follow the footsteps of our ancestors to do as they did, live or die without any criticisms whatever. For a long time I have followed the tenets of such teaching with unsatisfactory results until by reason and observation I have come to the conclusion that all so-called tracheal and lung disease are simply the effects following confused chemical action while in fermentation. Now I am satisfied that we know very little if anything of the attributes of the lungs and the importance of the duties that Nature has set apart for them to perform in animal life. But we do know from observation and experience that in all diseases of trachea and lungs we find variations of vertebrae and ribs from their perfectly normal position. By following this philosophy and practice we have been encouraged by the good results obtained to hope and be governed accordingly in the treatment of such diseases.

That lungs do generate gas is not debatable but for what purpose we are not able to say. We do know that much impurity is carried to the lungs by the venous system and from the receptaculum chyli and much explosive matter finds its way to the lungs and is exploded when it comes in contact with atmospheric air. Thus we have proof that much of the gas generated in the lungs by chemical action is used for vocal and musical purposes. Of the ability of the lung to supply the air that is used in singing and conversation we know very little. The fact is established by repeated demonstrations that the lungs alternate in receiving atmospheric air and expelling it after the chemical action of one lung is through its work. It is an easy matter now to demonstrate the fact that while the right lung is in action discharging its contents and resupplying itself with atmospheric air the left lung is silent and inactive and doing the laboratory work incumbent on it as a chemical separator of the impurities of the blood and other substances that are carried to the lungs for separation and purification to the degree of arterial blood.

How is this alternate action performed? The right pneumogastric nerve when it reaches the root of the right lung throws off two pulmonary plexuses, the anterior and posterior, whose functions are to rule and govern the lung according to Nature's plan and specification. That nerve is wholly independent of the nerve of the left lung which starts as the left pneumogastric from the brain, continues its course to the left lung, establishes two plexuses to rule and govern that lung which is also separate and apart from the right lung. This we know to be true. Thus we see by reason and prove by demonstration that one lung is silent while the other operates, and as soon as the operating lung has expelled the atmosphere and refills the other lung begins, expels and fills with atmosphere and soon as filled the opposite lung begins, discharges and refills. The action is perpetual during life; and that such is the case is not only reasonable, but is an absolute, demonstrable and demonstrated fact. With this fact demonstrated we feel that we now have a reliable philosophy by which to proceed in the treatment of lung diseases; this is an exception to all philosophies hitherto known. The treatment of lung diseases has been hitherto without reason in philosophy or satisfaction in results; death has been the rule.

To demonstrate alternate action of the lungs place a healthy person on the table on his back. Stand at his head and place your hands over the lungs. Have him exhale and inhale deeply. By the alternate movements of the chest wall beneath the hands you will soon find that one lung fills up with fresh air and retains that air until the other lung discharges the foul gases and refills with fresh air. This is what ordinarily occurs when the lungs are in action, but in order to generate enough gas for vocal purposes in continued speaking or in singing, both lungs are brought into action.

The lung has been a subject of great interest during all ages, but the philosophy of its action, and the results of its functioning have been overlooked and passed in silence. Whether it is a machine that executes a very important function in the animal life, and how it is made to act—whether both lungs move at once or one is silent for a time while the other acts in purifying, a portion of the blood—are questions we ask and desire some information upon, because no satisfactory information has ever been given by any author so far as we can learn. As engineers I propose that we treat this subject as if the lung were an engine and reason and work accordingly, because I am satisfied that this is the only school in which such truths are taught, learned, applied, demonstrated and made useful. Something is wrong or goes wrong in the action of the lungs previous to disease and death from lung trouble and we want to know where the break or friction started; how and why the lung has failed to perform its functioning. Then we will be better prepared to proceed to adjust to the normal and we will have a hope for restoring our patients to health. The normal and alternate action of both lungs must be maintained. It is reasonable that one lung cannot perform the duties of both lungs. If the left lung should become inactive and fail to do its chemical work of combustion and reducing impure substances to gas which it throws out, such deposits accumulate and form what is generally known as tubercles, both great and small. Then we have a cause of irritation, inflammation and destruction of the left lung, which is found by dissection of the consumptive's body to be more heavily laden with cheesy matter than the right lung. Thus the importance of the harmonious action of both lungs, or death by tuberculosis may be expected.

LUNG DISEASES PREVENTED
AND ERADICATED.

I speak only by comparison, when I speak to persons with whom I wish to exchange the benefits of reason, and I hope by such exchange of opinions to get the truth of any principle or law of Nature. Thus I compare what has been or is known of the law of cause and effect. In this case I will take lung diseases. The effect is well known to be death, but what is known of the first cause of the malady? If we judge by the number of cures or increase of deaths from consumption under old systems of treatment we are forced to say the cause or the cure of pulmonary tuberculosis has not been found. To this day all practitioners say by word and deed that they have failed to find either the cause or cure of consumption. The pathologists have killed dogs, doves and frogs; have analyzed blood, urine and saliva; they have labored hard without reporting either cause or cure. The chemist finds sugar, albumin, alkalies, acids and much that is not normal but his dying wife is a condemning witness to his knowledge of the cause that eats her as a hyena devours a rabbit. It is now left for the osteopath to see if he can find the cause of the lung's failure to do good work.

One writer says that a great per cent of nurses in lung sanitariums become consumptive and die; that in association with the patients, drinking, breathing, etc., they absorb the bacteria. I don't dispute this. It is very probable that it is true and that separation is necessary. The nurses should be careful not to inhale the foul breath from the consumptives nor drink after them, because if in poor health themselves from working too many hours, loss of sleep, etc., their physical condition will not resist the bacterial onslaught; then it would be reasonable to suppose that some of the attendants would be affected by the disease. I have been told that nearly forty per cent of the attendants contract tuberculosis, the reason for which I would attribute as much to exhaustion from overwork and lack of hygiene as to the theory of bacteria.

As an old soldier I made some observation on the field of battle where deadly smoke and poisonous gases from pistol, gun and cannon filled the air almost to the degree of suffocation. Two days after a fight between a regiment of General Price's men and a scout of two hundred of Fremont's men in which fifteen or twenty horses were killed, the decomposing gases were being thrown off from the dead bodies of the horses. We camped one day and two nights on the ground near these dead horses and breathed the gas and vapor coming from their bodies. As a result several hundred of my regiment were attacked in a few days with dysentery of a violent character. In cholera times we would have said Asiatic cholera. The horses were hauled away, but for several days there were other cases of dysentery because of having inhaled that gaseous poison. The poisonous gases were received by the lungs, taken up by the blood and distributed to the abdominal viscera and all the parts of the body. The result was dysentery.

Now what I want to emphasize is that a sanitarium for consumptives, where hundreds of diseased and dying people are brought together is just as poisonous as the spot of ground about the size of a sanitarium on which the dead horses lay. I do not recommend the bringing together of great numbers of persons whose lungs are throwing off deadly vapors and who constantly cough and spit the dead and decaying matter from the body.

When we have treated disease with success it has been because we knew the cause and proceeded accordingly; then the result was good. If a person is lame in one leg and not lame in the other, then one with the least knowledge of anatomy would direct his exploration to the lame leg to find the cause. He might look at the skin and if sound, he would pass to the bone; if not fractured but found sound, then he would go to the muscles; if sound he would pass to the blood vessels; if found normal he would go to the nerves; if abnormal by wound, disease or otherwise, he would seek the exact location. If a pin or nail were driven through and retained in the sciatic and he had found it, which in this case would be the location of the cause, he would pull that nail or pin out. If no nail or pin be found, but if he should find the sciatic or any other nerve suffering because of pressure from contracted muscles or any strain or hurt, he would remove that cause. If it is a dislocation of the hip joint, then put the hip back in the socket. If the condition has been one of only a few hours' or days' duration you may expect a speedy recovery. It is just as reasonable for one lung to be diseased and not the other as one leg and not the other; one eye and not the other; one ear and not the other. Thus you will see that your business is the treatment of the cause that has produced the disease.

When a person with lung disease comes to you for advice which to him may seem to be the final verdict as to his condition, I wish to impress on you and emphasize that what you say in his case is weighty far beyond your concept. Should you find any hope for his recovery and make that your report; like a thrill of lightning dipped in the sea of love, his vitality dances with joy. He is warmed up soul and body. But if you should be indiscreet enough in your report to remove every ray of hope, you have chilled the vital energy, you have silenced it, and the vegetable energies take possession of your patient and drag him with lightning speed to the valley of death. If you have any generalship you will evade anything like reporting that there is no hope for your patient. If you should analyze his substances and by your analysis see that there is no hope, be careful. Tell your patient that he is in such a condition that you wish to observe his case for a few days, weeks or months; that while man is alive he is not dead, and you hope to do him some good, though you and he both know his case is serious. Then if the patient concludes to stay and take a few days' treatment always come to him as though you wanted to do him all the good in your power, then he will be satisfied, and not break down in despair. This advice I offer to the young graduates. I think from long experience it is good, and wish you would govern yourselves accordingly. I am giving you the advice that is based upon my experience of many years.

I will give you the results of my many years' observation and experience as an osteopath. We will commence with our exploration for treatment by first listening to the cough and other manifestations of lung disease. We will then carefully examine the skin over the chest and see if it is cold. If so, address your attention to the nerves of temperature which are situated in each axilla passing from the neck down and under each scapula just above and behind the axillary arteries. When you have raised the pectoralis major muscle and gently slid your fingers back to the under surface of the scapula and on to the heat nerves above the axillary artery, nature responds to your touch for you have stimulated the nerves of temperature. Then the temperature will run up to the degree of natural heat, which is necessary to overcome the lower order known as the vegetable fermenting process. This by comparison you will understand as I will now give it to you, viz.; the animal ferment manifests itself by vital action, as when an egg is kept up to the temperature of ninety—eight degrees or above; the vital fermentation proceeds and the result is that it produces a living chicken. This, as you know, is the history and truth as proven by hens and incubators. You have had the hen egg for your consideration, now take the egg of the corn, which is the grain of corn, or a grain of wheat, or any vegetable seed from the vegetable world. It will sprout and grow when the ground only sustains a temperature of forty degrees or higher. Thus you understand the difference between animal and vegetable fermentation. The consumptive's lungs must be kept near the normal temperature, then the animal fermentation can proceed, and overcome the vegetable substances which are much more plentiful in the human body when its temperature is below normal.

Thus you see the importance of a normal temperature being maintained. It is of unlimited importance that you search every joint from the atlas to the coccyx and know that every vertebra is in its proper place, every rib in perfect articulation. Then the brain can dispense the necessary force to the heart to drive the blood into the aorta, both above and below the diaphragm. Then the intercostal branches that are thrown from the aorta are not obstructed or hindered in supplying the blood which is met by the internal mammary artery in the form of an anastomosis, which must be in perfect harmony and freedom of action, if you wish to sustain the animal above the vegetable temperature, which proves to be the successful general of death in croup, tonsillitis, diphtheria, pneumonia and all diseases of the glandular system of the body, none excepted. Hence, the importance of your wisdom and skill as an engineer, if you expect to succeed.

Now before leaving this subject, between the first and second ribs we have sensation; between the second and third ribs we have motion; between the third and fourth ribs we have nutrition; then we have between the fifth and sixth ribs sensation for the diaphragm; between the sixth and seventh ribs, motion for the diaphragm; between the seventh and eighth ribs we have nutrition for the diaphragm. This shows the importance of keeping the upper eight ribs and all the vertebrae in absolutely normal condition, or we may expect abnormal results from the heart or lungs.

LUNG DISEASES.

I have often asked the doctors of all schools of medicine to give me some light on diseases of the lungs. I have told them that I wanted to know the cause that produces the destructive effect known to be eating the life out of millions of people every twelve months. I have asked the doctors for fifty years to give me the cause of the trouble, not the effect. I know the effect—dead folks. They have told me what some pathologist says he has found in the sputum that was different from a well man's sputum. I would tell the doctor that his story was nice, but I wanted to know just the exact spot that I could go to and learn why one person was free and another person a slave and his end was death. Then the doctor would tell me that whisky was good for tuberculosis. I have had such evasive bosh for lo these many years, without one jot or tittle of proof that the doctor had ever dreamed of the cause of any disease of the lungs. If we want to know why, let us follow the blood from the heart as it journeys through the great and small arteries. Let us follow with the microscope of observation until we find a halt at some organ, muscle, bone or skin. Halt and stay until we know just what the result is. If that blood curdles and separates into many parts then we will know that a deadly chemical action has stopped the work of draining, and fermentation has set in and deposits will pile up in that part of the system and produce death as far as the deposits go. What have medical schools done for consumptives more than to follow them to their graves? The doctor would save them if he could, but he has lung disease himself, doses, drinks and dies. His brother doctor also has pulmonary disease, drinks, dopes and dies; goes to his grave and leaves no hope for others because he never went farther than his morphine and whisky bottle. His pathology taught him nothing of cause; he lived and died proving to the world the insufficiency of drugs and drink. He could see no cause for lung disease in the fermentation of blood with its deadly deposits in the system. This was all a blank to him.

All methods and systems of healing have proven to be failures in combating diseases of the lungs, and are so acknowledged and accepted, not only by many of the best authors, but proven to be so by the continual and undiminished funeral processions. I feel no timidity in agreeing with the sages of medicine that such is the case, and I ask for a more reliable compass by which we may be conducted to some system of philosophy that will open out for us the cause or causes that produce pulmonary diseases. The prevailing systems have fought manfully. They have failed. They have also universally combated effects. They have analyzed the substances thrown from the lungs while yet alive; they have also analyzed the lungs after death and have acted upon their conclusions, but have not diminished the mortality. With all these methods practiced, and proven failures, we feel free to hunt farther and deeper, with a hope that we may obtain some knowledge of the cause or causes, that is trustworthy and practicable. We know that inflammation of the lungs generally begins in the right side, and is known as pneumonia, also in post mortems we find the left lung containing tubercular deposits of cheesy matter. We find abnormal conditions of the pleurae local and general, high up and low down. What evidence have we that the pleura is not responsible for the abnormal condition of the lung after having been exposed to atmospheric changes? We know that the pleura is well supplied with nerves and blood, we know that it has much to do with the healthy or unhealthy condition of the lung. Why is the lung divided into two sections or divisions, with three lobes on the right, two on the left? Is this a provision of Nature to receive the atmospheric air all on the right side when the temperature is very low and cold?

The right lung is situated in the right side of the thorax and it has as you know, three lobes. The left lung is situated in the left side, and has two lobes. Each lung extends just above the first rib. The left lung extends as low down as the ninth rib. The right lung as low down as the eighth rib. They are in separate sacs known as the pleurae. They are provided with separate nerves starting at the brain and extending to the root of the lungs where they form plexuses, both front and rear, which are distributed over and through the lungs in such a manner as to accommodate every demand of the lungs in their action, whether that action be separate or united. These nerves are known as the pneumogastric nerves.

I give this that the student of this philosophy may freshen his memory on the points to which his exploration for cause of disease is to be directed. When we reason about the cause or causes of lung disturbances we will be confined to the nerve and blood supply in which the lung is directly interested. If that lung is dependent for its force on the pneumogastric nerve, and that nerve is dependent on the brain and spinal cord for its own strength and nourishment, we must know that that nerve from the brain to the lung and from the lung to the heart is absolutely clear of all impingements. Then we may expect normal force and action. If that lung is dependent on the heart and the nerves that accompany the blood vessels from the heart to the lung for nourishment, then we must be careful to know that there is no impingement by spine or ribs that would interfere with perfect nerve and blood supply to the heart, thence to the lung, without which perfect supply we have no foundation to hope for good results. If the first, second, third, fourth or even down as low as the ninth rib should show any variation from correct articulation, you are not warranted in stopping until you have adjusted the rib to the vertebra and that vertebra to other sections of the spine.

In any lung disease, without exception, you cannot be too exacting in your exploration and the work of readjusting to the normal, because impingements on the pneumogastric or any other nerve that adds to the action and support of the lung, often produce paralysis of a part or the whole of a lobe, or all of the lobes of that lung. Thus you have congestion, stagnation, fermentation, precipitation and deposits of casein or cheesy matter in the cells and cellular membranes, which is the beginning of the progressive action of tuberculosis or pulmonary consumption. Keep your eyes open and see that from the occiput to the tenth rib on either side there is no interference with any nerve pertaining to the trachea, lung or pleura, because I believe on this foundation is your hope for the recovery of your patient.

Remember this, that while punching, wringing and twisting your patient who has lung trouble, unless you have a thorough knowledge of the location of the lung, its form, its nerve and blood supply, you are doing your patient no good, and yourself a great deal of harm by your failure to give relief. When you have correctly adjusted the framework, also the nerve and blood supply, you will often be surprised to see the patient discharge half a pint of corruption at one time, which is a strong evidence that you have adjusted the recuperating power of the lungs and the machinery is unobstructed. They will clean out deposits and repair injuries by cicatrizing and closing up the cavity from whence issues this pus, and you may expect to see your patient return to good health, enjoyment of life and ability to follow his usual avocation. I think there is hope for the consumptive if the case is taken before the lungs are too far gone. I have practiced on this line with good success for thirty years and am gratified at the happy results that Nature has been able to give. When all is normal in structure, good results can be expected.

Treatment.—Diseases of the thorax are those of the heart, lungs, pleura and pericardium. In treating the organs of the chest we must be governed by the nerve and blood supply of the whole chest from the first to the tenth dorsal, because in this area is the heart which must have blood and force to supply the whole system of the thorax, also all the organs of that system. The heart must have all of its blood-vessels and their nerves clear from obstructions of any kind or it will fail to do good work. A feeble heart cannot do good work. You must keep its blood and nerves strong and well fed or it cannot pull its load. Thus you have work to do from the brain to the tenth dorsal. Your work is on both spine and ribs, from the first to the tenth rib. Generally you will find the fifth and sixth ribs on the left side close together, shutting off the intercostal artery; you will often find this is the case in palpitation of the heart. Much of the labor of the heart is to force the blood through the intercostal arteries to the mammary connection which is by anastomosis. You find intercostal freedom gives relief in palpitation of the heart.

I think bony lesions are responsible for much of the trouble in the thorax. I mean by bony lesions a sufficient strain or dislocation to produce pressure and obstruct the normal discharge of nerve and blood supply. Sometimes we find them squeezed so closely as to produce adhesive inflammation and bony union. Any osteopath who is posted in anatomy, by dissection or otherwise, knows this to be true of the bony system of the thorax. The osteopath of practice and skill knows and has demonstrated to his own satisfaction that when he adjusts the spine and ribs, the heart acts normally. To him this is not theory but a truth of his own demonstration. When the blood starts from the heart to the head he knows that if it goes through to the brain and if the venous return is good it will do its work properly and the report will be "all is well." If not, it is impossible to do the work. Thus we must explore for and keep the track open, then the organs of the head will be supplied. The same with the neck; the same with the lungs. Keep the gates of life all open. If you do not the bad results proclaim a failure to find and treat the cause.

PNEUMONIA.

Definition.—Any disease of the lung characterized by exudation into the alveoli and bronchioles resulting in consolidation and functional uselessness of the affected area. There are two main clinical forms of pneumonia, viz., croupous or lobar pneumonia and catarrhal or lobular pneumonia, which are entirely distinct diseases. See these forms below. When the term pneumonia is employed alone or without any qualification, croupous or lobar pneumonia is generally understood.

Croupous Pneumonia.—Lobar pneumonia, an acute febrile disease caused by the toxins of the Diplococcus pneumoniae or Micrococcus lanceolatus. There are three stages of pneumonia: Stage of engorgement or congestion: the affected lung is distended, of a red color, firmer, and crepitates less than normal lung tissue. Red hepatization or consolidation: the affected portion becomes solid, brownish in color, resembling normal liver tissue; alveoli and smaller bronchi are filled with solid exudation. Gray hepatization and resolution or purulent infiltration; affected portion becomes gray by the decoloration of the blood globules; infiltration or absorption takes place; gangrene or calcareous encapsulation may occur. Predisposing causes: Age, mostly under five years, then between 20 and 40, and after 60; poverty, intemperance, and sudden changes of temperature; Exciting causes: Exposure to changes of temperature; atmospheric conditions. Symptoms: Distinct chills (violent for one-half or two hours); these are absent only in old people after 70; prostration; pain underneath the nipple of affected side; increased respirations, more than thirty per minute; dyspnoea, cough; mucous expectoration at first, afterward becoming gelatinous, viscid, tenacious, yellow or brick-dust color; countenance is flushed; temperature, 102-105 F. Catarrhal pneumonia has in general the same stages and symptoms as croupous; restrained movement, normal vocal fremitus, slight dulness, crackling sounds heard at the end of inspiration; crepitant rales heard in the first twelve or twenty-four hours. Crepitant rale is a characteristic sign of first stage of pneumonia. Second stage: Inspection—expansive movements are diminished on the affected and increased on the healthy side. Palpation—as a rule, increased vocal fremitus. Percussion—marked dulness. Auscultation—

bronchial breathing; bronchophony. Third stage: Physical signs in early part of this stage are the same as those of the second stage. Rude (or bronchovesicular) respiration, subcrepitant and crepitant rales. Prognosis is bad in the very young or very old, alcoholics, or those debilitated by pre-existing disease.

—Dunglison.

On prognosis and treatment Dunglison's old edition contains the following:

Prognosis.—In young children and old persons almost always fatal. Double pneumonia generally fatal.

Treatment.—In vigorous and undoubtedly healthy individuals, with elevated temperature and high pulse, flushed surface and marked dyspnoea, bleeding has been resorted to by some advocates; rest in bed; liquid food, milk, eggs; for pain and cough, opium; for high temperature, quinia. If the heart is feeble stimulants, alcohol or carbonate of ammonium, digitalis; nutritious diet, and, when the violence of the inflammation has been subdued, counter-irritation, etc. Chronic pneumonia sometimes succeeds the acute form, or it may occur accidentally; must be managed on general principles, and counter-irritants of all kinds are indicated.

—Dunglison.

For many years the medical writers have tried to unfold the mysteries of pneumonia but have failed. I think it is well enough for the mechanic to offer a few thoughts that will point out the friction that produces that condition of the lungs. The reader who desires to obtain some knowledge of what it is and what has produced it, finds nothing satisfactory written by any author up to the present date.

Pneumonia, enlarged tonsils, inflammation of the trachea or of the entire pulmonary system, according to any writings that I can find, are just as little understood as is their treatment, and it proves itself as deficient as though nothing had been written. The methods of treatment are just as uncertain as the course of a vessel would be without a compass to guide it. The medical doctors have tried the old, the new, the hot, the cold, the sedative, the stimulant, and the various kinds of gases, but the result has been the same, and I think it always will be until the engineer who is acquainted with all the parts of the human body comes and adjusts the machinery. He realizes that there is friction in the pulmonary system or in the region of the thorax, and that it must be found before he can proceed intelligently to give his patient relief. He proceeds to remove from any point between the base of the skull and the coccyx, any pressure sufficient to produce a constriction of the nervous system or obstruct the flow of venous blood to the heart. Such retention is followed by stagnation, fermentation and destructive decomposition.

We must remember that a chemical process soon begins in the venous blood when not in motion, as it is far from being pure. The change continues until the blood becomes poisonous in quality and an overplus in quantity, engorging the lungs with impure blood, making it impossible for them to separate the impure from the pure, and to return a sufficient quantity of arterial blood, having the constructive ability of a healthy circulation. The engineer sees pneumonia as an effect, the cause being a tightening of all parts of the entire system. To the osteopath who understands the human body as the engineer does his engine, all the mysteries disappear. The law of cause and effect is understood, and he governs himself accordingly. He may expect his patient to get well if he has taken the case reasonably early.

When it is proved that the competent engineer of the human body is a failure in the treatment of diseases of the lungs, the plurae, the tonsils and all the organs of the respiratory tract, then we will run up the white flag of defeat and join the medical world and cry aloud that our system also is a failure.

How is the inflammation resulting from imperfect venous drainage or failure of the blood to properly return from the pleura or lung supposed to be produced? In such cases the arteries are abnormally active and the supply is greater than the consumption because the venous system does not appropriate it. Thus we have congestion simply by blood being retained in the venous system when it should have passed on. Had the venous system drained the parts normally then we would have no overplus to go through the process of fermentation to the degree of pus.

By this philosophy the reader can easily see what has caused the whole abnormal condition found before and after death. The chemist says something; the pathologist says much; and the microscopist says a great deal. But to the osteopath the results are due to stagnation and fermentation; and to him such voluminous stories are of but little if any benefit in the successful treatment of lung diseases. The microscope, the thermometer, the chemical laboratory all together have never given us a single trustworthy remedy, for the reason that they do not go back to the cause, which is, in all cases, obstruction to venous and arterial normal action.

You say "the patient must have relief from this suffering. How are we to proceed?" The doctor of medicine has no hesitation in the free administration of drugs. We ask the doctor what effect he expects by the morphine and other palliative drugs, hot bags, etc. He has no hesitancy in informing you with the wise look of a philosopher, that he wants and is laboring to give ease instead of pain. This is the information you obtain from your question. From him you get no idea that a variation of spine, vertebrae, ribs or muscles produces the obstruction and causes the condition that confuses the vital action of the pulmonary system.

Let us reason a little farther. If you have had a boil or any deposit of pus that gave you great misery, do you remember what followed the act of letting the pus out? Did you not get relief? That pus was not hurting you, because it was dead. It was the nerves that hurt. They were impinged by the deposit of blood that had gone through the process of fermentation and so had piled up the obstructing bulk. Now if we know the anatomy of nerve and blood supply to and from the lungs the door is wide open and we can see the cause or causes that produce obstruction of venous blood, and we know just what to do to give relief. If we do not know our business we will call in a medical doctor who administers morphine. When morphine enters the body it takes possession, and says to the blood in the venous system, "Keep still!"; and to the cellular system and excretory ducts, "Be quiet!"; and they are still as far as misery is concerned. But during the quietness vegetable fermentation proceeds with its work, carries on decomposition and the congestion becomes general instead of local and death scores another victory.

Now let me tell you that just as letting the pus out of the boil relieved you, so when you let the blood pass on from any part of the body in which there is congestion you relieve the misery in that part. If you slip a rib or any joint up, down, back or forward, you obstruct the nerve or blood supply, or drainage in the venous system and some disturbance will result.

Etiology.—Pneumonia is a condition which is the effect of atmospheric changes, especially on patients who have become debilitated from any cause. The result of such changes is a shock so far reaching in its effects that all of the

110

structures of the body are disturbed thereby. The nerves become irritated, then the vessels carrying the blood and lymph contract, then the muscles, until there is attained the degree of general contracture, and the nerves, veins and arteries are placed on a strain in their effort to carry out normal functioning. The lymphatic system in its contracted condition fails to take up its usual supply of lymph for delivery through the thoracic duct to the veins for the heart. Consequently there is a lowering of the nutritive quality of the blood as well as the rate of circulation. As a result the blood stagnates, ferments and soon becomes overcharged with decomposing substances robbing the seeds of life of their constructive power. The lungs become irritated, the venous drainage is hindered by the contractures, the capacity of the lungs is diminished, they are unable to take in oxygen in normal quantities, and the breath becomes labored, short and quick. I want to emphasize that we must have a good nerve and blood supply to the pleurae when we treat the lungs.

Treatment.—With the fact demonstrated that venous blood must pass on, up and through the azygos major and minor veins and other veins that perfect the drainage of the venous blood from the spinal and costal areas of the abdomen and thorax, we will ask you to refresh your memory by consulting your anatomy on nerve and blood supply of the whole spine, particularly that from the occiput to the diaphragm. You will see that the azygos veins are three in number and receive the venous blood from the dorsal and lateral thoracic walls. The bronchial veins accompany the bronchial arteries, only part of whose blood they return, that distributed to the smaller bronchi entering the pulmonary veins. They pass out at the back of the root of the lung and enter the upper end of the vena azygos major on the right side and the left upper azygos or the left superior intercostal vein on the left side. The intercostal veins, the main tributaries of the azygos veins, receive large dorsal branches from the muscles of the back, the dorsal spinal plexus and the spinal canal.

I have successfully treated many cases of pneumonia, both lobar and pleuritic, by correcting the ribs at their spinal articulations. If I find much cutting pain in lung and pleura, I carefully palpate over the upper ribs of the side on which the pain is located. I usually find the sixth, seventh and eighth ribs pushed above or below or twisted upon the transverse processes thus closing up the intercostal veins by pressure and disturbing the vaso motors to the lungs. I carefully adjust the misplaced ribs and if a cough continues to annoy the patient, explore higher up for a displaced first, second, third or fourth rib and correct any variations found. Such variations may cause a tightening of the clavicle pressing down on branches of the pneumogastric nerve as they pass under it. Carefully adjust ribs and clavicle and the cough will cease, if taken in time. When the ribs are adjusted and the blood and nerve supply freed from pressure, the fever generally goes down and ease will follow.

Carefully examine the spine where the renal nerves issue from the Spinal cord. Adjust all variations from normal. Give close attention to the eleventh and twelfth dorsal vertebrae. You may expect to find heavily contracted lumbar muscles which produce a drawing together of the spinous articulations from the lower dorsal to the sacrum. I think the contraction of these muscles is because the kidneys are not normally taking up and passing off urine and other fluids through the bladder. Be careful to know that you have brought the base of the fifth lumbar far enough forward to let the nerves that are irritated by the contraction of the lumbar muscles free. This irritation is suspending a free action of the sacral nerves. We must have this fluid passed through the kidneys; hence the importance of careful examination and correct adjustment of the region of the spine which I have pointed out.

Now you have prepared your kidney to excrete and your bladder to receive. Go higher up the spine and know that the atlas is properly, adjusted, and also each and all of the joints of the neck. All the ribs and articulations of the upper dorsal must be absolutely correct, then you can expect a better circulation of the blood. It will not circulate normally if there is any impingement on the tenth nerves. They must be without irritation. We must have freedom of the nerve and blood circulation in the axilla also. We want no stagnation or stoppage in the axilla because it should keep up a continuous return of the venous blood which belongs to the whole axillary system; for in pneumonia the heart drives the blood in the arteries with increased force, but if the venous return is delivered as fast as the arterial is given, then we have a reduction of the excitability of the axillary system.

Be careful, after exploring and adjusting the upper spine and ribs, to know that the atlas is in perfect position. Travel on down from atlas to seventh, and know that all cervical vertebrae are in normal position. Be careful to draw the inferior maxilla forward and the atlas backward in order to secure free flow of blood and nerve force to and from the brain. From the brain we get our forces

112

and from the heart we get our supply, and in order to get good results the channels from brain and heart must have freedom from irritation. My experience for many years has been such that I can say this philosophy is true; and I hope that every osteopath will go deep enough into the science to see that it is, and then let his work stand as a voucher.

PULMONARY TUBERCULOSIS.

Definition of Tuberculosis.—Disease caused by the growth and development of the tubercle bacillus. It is characterized usually by the presence of the peculiar formations called tubercles. It may affect any organ or tissue in the body, but is particularly prone to attack the lungs in adults, the intestines and mesenteric glands in children; the bones and joints are also frequent seats of tuberculous disease, especially in children.

—Dunglison.

Pulmonary Tuberculosis.—Tuberculosis of the lungs.

—Dunglison.

Tuberculosis is an effect following inhibition of the nerve and blood supply which results in retention, stagnation and fermentation and in producing a cheesy matter which is deposited in the cellular tissue of the whole pulmonary system.

By many Dr. Osler is considered the best of the present day writers, but after carefully perusing all his writings on pulmonary tuberculosis, I conclude that while he has found the system out of running order, and a friction set up in some part of the body producing a confusion the result of which is tuberculosis, if I understand him he does not say a single word that gives light on the cause of this abnormal condition. He quotes the usual number of authors and makes free use of a vocabulary of technicalities, and leaves us to understand that he knows but little if anything of the cause producing the malady. For many years I have been a faithful reader of medical authors, ancient and modern. I have followed them through their books, laboratories, rooms of counsel—great and small, their diagnosis and treatment; and so far as consumption is concerned, they agree that it has done, does, and will do its work of destruction. But in their combat with this disease the best ammunition they use is a blank cartridge. This is the verdict reported by the great jury of the graveyard.

Etiology.—When an author writes on tuberculosis, typhoid fever or any other disease and closes his argument by saying "we do not know the cause or causes that have produced this disease," we all, from the ordinary reasoner to the greatest philosopher, naturally raise the question, can we be guided by such writing, notwithstanding that the author is honest enough to acknowledge he has failed to obtain any information on that subject? The man who is able to reason will ask such questions as these: Do you ever have a sour stomach? Can we have a fermentation and sourness of the lymph in the lymphatics of the superficial fascia? Can you smell that sour odor coming through the skin from the superficial fascia? Can the lymph in the lymphatics of the pleurae and lungs ferment and throw off a sour smell? If it can, haven't you a fact concerning tuberculosis? The answer is yes.

He will ask other questions: does the lymph in the lymphatics of the fascia and the venous system ever sour? What is the condition of the lymph and other fluids when they have gone through the process of fermentation from sugar to acids? Does milk coagulate and form hard substances commonly known as curd or clabber? Does that curd fall down or does it float in the watery fluids of the milk? If the lymph and other fluids sour and clot in the fascia of the human system, and if this cheesy substance is carried to the lungs and fails to pass through the capillary circulation but piles up and forms tubercles, haven't you something to guide your mental compass beyond the imaginary and unsatisfactory stories of the tubercle bacilli, and to show you that tuberculosis is the result of the sour condition of the lymphatics of the universal fascia?

Does your consumptive's breath and perspiration smell sour? Does his urine coagulate? Do the branches of the aorta have any obstruction that would hinder the intercostal arteries from passing their blood through the intercostal system that unites with the mammary artery? If the harmony of blood action is suspended will this blood stagnate and sour? Will the deposits of cheese be the result? These are the questions that pass through the mechanical reasoner's mind. He is sure to have to repeat his question until he has yes or no for an answer, also a demonstration that vouches for his knowledge of the cause that produces the effect known as tuberculosis. If this philosophy be true, then much of the mystery of tuberculosis will disappear and give room for demonstrated truth.

I use simple English. I say bone, brain or buttermilk, and try to use such plain terms that any intelligent person will know what I mean. I want to be understood when I say that previous to tubercular formations the blood or milk of life sours, coagulates, and dumps its wads into the lungs or other parts of the body. I hope to speak in such plain English that the laity will know the difference between scholastic delusion and truth.

Suppose a boy kills cats and throws them under the bed in which you sleep, then decomposition sets in and makes you sick. Would you spend your time reading dietetics or would you remove the cats? Make the application; the pneumogastric nerve, the intercostals and the whole pulmonary system represent the cat-killing boy. In all consumptives that I have examined and treated in the last thirty-five years the intercostal nerves, arteries and veins were inhibited by ribs which were thrown from their proper articulation with the transverse processes of the spine. The ribs I usually find affected are from the first to the fourth and on down to the eighth on either side.

What is the difference between the healthy and the unhealthy lung? We will try to answer this question as a mechanic. When we have disease of the lungs I think it is reasonable to conclude that by some process the lungs have become the excretory dumping ground for the system; whereas normally the system should dump the waste matter into the bladder, the bowels, the skin as well as the lungs. When the lungs do their normal part as one of the excreting organs, and the skin, the bowels and the kidneys do their part also, and the brain is uninterrupted in its function then we have no such thing as lung disease. But when we have a perversion of the excretory system and the burden is all thrown upon the lungs then we have congestion, a piling up, a fermentation, a suppuration, a decomposition of the substances of the entire body. The lungs become exhausted, the fluids sour, and cheesy matter is separated from and deposited in the cellular system of the lungs in such quantities as to congest, irritate and inflame, and its decomposition keeps up this perpetual issue of pus or matter from the lungs.

I reason that if the system when perverted from the normal makes a dumping ground of the lungs, that they very soon become overpowered and exhausted. The machine is changed from one of vital construction to one in which there is a consuming fire of destruction whose object is to burn up the waste matter, get it out of the way and give the vital fluids and forces a chance to leave the abnormal and return to their original normal condition. Hence I reason that when the normal excretory system is able to excrete impurities from the body as fast as they are generated, we have not only a hope but a certainty of giving relief and cure in what is commonly known as consumption, especially when the case is taken and treated before the period of collapse appears. Otherwise destruction of the whole body will be the effect of the poisonous compounds which take the place of the normal juices and fluids of all the organs of the whole system.

Now I have "sized up" the enemy and brought him in line of battle. You know his strength, his skill and how you must proceed to combat this enemy—pulmonary tuberculosis—who has never yet known the meaning of the word surrender.

Treatment.—In giving you a mechanic's philosophy and method of treatment of lung diseases, as I understand them, I will draw your attention to the importance of the nerve and blood supply of the pleurae and lungs; also to the excretory structures of the body—the lungs, the fascia, the skin, the kidneys, the bowels; and to the brain as the chief source of all action. The engineer in charge of any machine to apply force by water, steam or electricity is very careful to know that all parts of the machine are in good order for perfect action, and sufficient to execute the work designed. Hence he examines his furnace, his boilers, his pipes of supply, his pipes of drainage, mud valves, and so forth.

He knows that if he shows intelligence and his machinery does good work he will hold his place. If not the boss-workman will discharge him for incompetency. The desired results will fail to appear because of this mechanic's ignorance. His work is to cut lumber, make flour or to do whatever that machine is intended for. He knows it is incumbent on him to know all parts belonging to the machine, to inspect and to keep every part in its proper place, cleaned and oiled, to fire up, turn on the steam and see that all is in good order; then good work is the result.

Now I will say no more to the skilled osteopath than to tell him to begin with his work on the consumptive patient at the neck, and explore and adjust the atlas and all joints of the spine and ribs from the head to the coccyx. There is no use for me to tell you how to adjust an atlas if you know your business, and your papers and your diploma all testify that you do. Now prove your worthiness by your work. You must have action, excretion of the skin, so fetch on the nerve and blood supply for both fascia and skin. This is the true compass to find the boy that killed the cats.

As you have adjusted the head with the neck and supplied the skin and fascia with the necessary blood supply and nerve action, we will take the next system, the lungs and the pleurae, and see that nothing interferes with their normal action. Thus you will see that a careful examination and adjustment of the spine and ribs is absolutely necessary in order to make sure that all joints are in place at every point.

Now as we have normal action of the pneumogastric and all other nerves relating to the lungs, before leaving this division we will ask: Have you carefully explored and adjusted that part of the spine and ribs that by malposition will in any way interfere with the normal action of the heart? If so we will pass on to that part of the spine which throws off the excretory nerves to the liver, the spleen, the kidneys, the ureters, the bladder and all of the pelvic viscera.

As I have so often shown you how to adjust the whole spinal system below the diaphragm for good and wholesome action both in secreting and in excreting, I will say no more on the excretory system for you surely know the importance of it and will do your work accordingly. Be very sure you have the clavicles in their proper position. Also the manubrium must be brought to its normal place on the gladiolus or there will be an irritation of the respiratory system. Give the lungs a chance to do their part and see that your patient gets plenty of good fresh air, judicious exercise on foot or on horseback and plenty of good plain wholesome nourishing food, for energy is necessary to throw off all impure deposits. Continual shaking of the abdomen by coughing and hacking makes the bowels sore and inflamed, and they are then unable to secrete pure chyle for the nutrition of the lungs and other tissues. This soreness of the bowels goes on to dysentery, which is the terminal complication of consumption, and this fact shows that the bowels need supporting; therefore, feed the colon with gruel as in typhoid fever. In these cases fill the colon three times a week. All cases of lung trouble, if taken in reasonable time, can be cured.

ASTHMA.

Definition.—A chronic disease characterized by great difficulty of breathing, recurring at intervals, accompanied by wheezing sounds, a sense of constriction in the chest, and sometimes cough and expectoration. It is frequently hereditary. In some cases respiration is universally puerile during the attack. In the spasmodic form the respiratory murmur is very feeble or absent, and in all forms percussion elicits a clear pulmonary sound. The disease generally consists in a spasmodic constriction of the smaller bronchial ramifications.

—Dunglison.

Etiology—Some persons have what we all know and what the medical doctors have defined as asthma. We all know the fuss made and the trouble experienced in breathing by the asthmatic. All authors agree that they know but little about the cause or cure of this distressing condition. The medical doctors send their patients to the mountains, advise them to smoke some kind of weed or drug, and so on. There are some who claim that asthma is hereditary. Thus ends the story.

I will give the osteopathic student the benefit and result of my experience, observation and success in the treatment of asthmatic patients, both young and old. I reasoned that there must be a mechanical cause for all this fuss and trouble in breathing, because sometimes the patient would breathe naturally, which showed me that at that time the lungs executed their function normally.

As a mechanic I examined the union of ribs with the spine, and in many cases, particularly on the right side at about the fifth, sixth, seventh and eighth, some or all of these ribs were off, under or above the transverse processes of the vertebrae. Also the muscles were in an abnormal condition in this and other parts of the spine, lower down and higher up. Many cases of asthma show renal disturbances with abnormal conditions of the spine in that region. Following the adjustment of these abnormal conditions to their natural positions came relief and cure. When by some jolt, wrench or strain the ribs were again pushed up or down (more often up), this would result in the same fuss and difficulty in breathing as before.

Treatment.—I sometimes treat asthmatic patients while they are standing up in the doorway, and at other times on the table. I place the back against the jamb of the door holding both shoulder blades squarely and firmly in place against the jamb. I then take my patient's right arm with my right hand, place my left hand under and back of the arm pit or axilla, carrying my fingers along the spine two or three inches above the lower border of the scapula so as to get my fingers on to the offending rib or ribs at their articulation with the transverse processes of the vertebrae. Now I raise the arm up strongly, pressing my right shoulder against the patient's sternum, bringing the arm straight up, high and parallel with the spine and head. While in that position I throw the arm backward and firmly hold it up until I can pull the rib well up or down and in place. Now I draw the arm across or back of the head strongly and return the arm to the side, keeping my fingers firmly against the offending rib until it finds its place. Then taking hold at the elbow give it a strong forceful push up in order to loosen all muscles and ligaments that could hold down a rib below the transverse process of the vertebra.

After this is done I turn my patient's breast toward the door-jamb and beginning at the eighth rib, with my thumbs I push up or down all ribs, even to the first, and know that every articulation is absolutely correct, When you know that this part of the work is absolutely normal then keep your hands off the patient for at least one week, unless there is no abatement of the asthmatic condition, which has never occurred in my osteopathic practice and with this method of treatment. I have never had a case that was not relieved, and many of them almost instantaneously. On two or three occasions I have had to treat my patient on the second day following the attack, but on examination I found that I had not brought the rib up to its normal articulation.

If we have followed this method carefully with our asthmatic patient and have done a good job with ribs and spine, and the breathing continues to be normal, let the patient alone in that condition for a week and give the parts there a chance to get over the spinous and intercostal irritation. I want to emphasize to you each and all that if you pull and haul your asthmatic patient every day, you will surely fail. For a day or two after treatment some of my patients report that they have coughed up as much as one pint of ropy substance in twelve hours. This is evidence that the lung is again beginning to do good work.

Keep your patient under close observation for two or three months and should the asthmatic condition recur you may know that some one of the ribs has dropped again, or there has been a return of some of the abnormal conditions which produced it. During the past thirty years I have treated many asthmatics and have had no failures except one or two which were far gone with tuberculosis. In regard to diet I have no advice to give, further than to allow such patients to eat what they want of good plain nutritious food.

I have had a number of cases which the medical doctors had sent to the mountains, but without avail; others who had been smoked with jimson weed and dosed with various preparations and who were then declared hopeless and were suffering a good deal when they reached me. I treated them after this method, and they are now enjoying freedom from asthma. By this method I have successfully treated patients of all ages and of both sexes, in the acute and also in the chronic stage. I want to emphasize that you need not be particular about any one method, but you must know that the ribs have been taken from the abnormal and left in their normal position.

LECTURE ON THE HEART.

Definition of Heart.—Azygous muscle, of an irregularly pyramidal shape, situated obliquely and a little to the left side in the chest; resting on the diaphragm by one of its surfaces; suspended by its base from the great vessels; free and movable in the rest of its extent, and surrounded by the pericardium. The right side of the body of the heart is thin and sharp, the left is thick and round. It is hollow within, and contains four cavities, two of which, with thinner and less fleshy walls, receive the blood from the lungs and the rest of the body, and pour it into two others with thick and very fleshy parietes, which send it to the lungs and to every part of the body. Of these cavities, the former are called auricles, the latter ventricles. The right auricle and right ventricle form the pulmonic or right or anterior heart; the left auricle and ventricle, the systemic, corporeal, left, or aortic heart. In the adult these are totally distinct from each other, being separated by a partition, the septum cordis. Into the right auricle the venae cavae, superior and inferior, and the coronary vein open. The pulmonary artery arises from the right ventricle (see Conus arteriosus); the four pulmonary veins open into the left auricle, and the aorta arises from the left ventricle.

The mean weight of the adult heart is, according to Bouillaud, from eight to nine ounces. The heart is covered externally by a very thin, membranous reflection from the pericardium. The muscular structure of the heart is much thicker in the parietes of the ventricles than in those of the auricles. Its cavities are lined by a very delicate membrane, the endocardium, continuous with the inner membrane of the arteries as regards the left cavities, and with that of the veins as regards the right. Its arteries, the coronary, arise from the commencement of the aorta. Its nerves proceed chiefly from the pneumogastric and the cervical ganglions of the great sympathetic. The heart is the great agent of the circulation; by its contraction the blood is sent over every part of the body. When the ear is applied to the chest a dull, lengthened sound is heard, synchronous with the arterial pulse. This is instantly succeeded by a sharp, quick sound, like that of the valve of a bellows or the lapping of a dog, and this is followed by a period of repose. Different views are entertained as to the causes of these sounds of the heart, which are evidently produced by contraction of the ventricles and consequent tension of the auriculoventricular valves by reflux of blood against the semilunar valves, etc. The word lubb-dup conveys a notion of the two sounds. The beating or impulse of the heart, heart stroke, apex beat, against the parietes of the chest, is mainly caused by the systole of the heart tending to project it forward.

The valves of the heart are situated as follows: Aortic, opposite the third intercostal space on the left side, close to the sternum; pulmonary, opposite the junction of the third rib with the sternum; mitral, opposite the third intercostal space, an inch to the left of the sternum aortic, behind the middle of the sternum at the level of the fourth rib.

—Dunglison.

"Give honor to whom honor is due." I think this old adage will apply to the heart as appropriately as to any person. Why should we give honor to the heart? The human heart is a most trustworthy servant. I say trustworthy because it does all its work to the full measure of skilled perfection. It is the dwelling place of the machinist of all known and unknown perfection in the art of constructing that which none other can construct. It constructs its own habitation, selects its own local dwelling place and manufactures all of its constructing machinery. It manufactures from crude material all substances of every grade and kind with which to construct the machinery of all divisions of its own manufacturing laboratory. In all departments of the chemical laboratory it proceeds to construct the organs and divisions of life out of which come the products of perfect purity—the superstructure known as the human body.

With this fact established in the mind of the operator it is much easier for him to proceed with his work successfully. Then he proceeds, knowing that the nerve and blood supply are absolutely necessary in the economy of all nature. And when he wishes a change from the abnormal or diseased condition to the normal or healthy he knows just how to proceed to explore from the affected part back to headquarters—from any extremity or division back to the heart—and in doing this he will find the cause that has produced the disease that he wishes to abate. He will find one of three conditions; interference with the nerve supply, the arterial supply, or the venous return, due to pressure or wound. This is not at all debatable. It is an absolute truth, self evident and demonstrable by him who knows what this machine is and knows what will cause a clogging hindrance. It matters not whether the obstruction be in foot, neck, arm, head, abdomen or back. This law is absolute, and the heart is the chief commissary of supply, and the nerve is the quartermaster that executes all orders from the heart.

We have reasons to believe the heart is one of the most important organs in the system. The first effort we see in fetal life is to construct the heart after forming a little cup, cell or chamber in which we always find a small amount of blood that proceeds on and on until it has formed a heart sufficient to receive and propel the blood in various directions. This small heart center seems to be endowed with a mind to foresee the necessity of blood-vessels. By its own energy it creates and locates nerves over which the forces for the construction of arteries and veins are conducted. Then it proceeds to form a being which it has the power and intelligence to construct with all the attributes necessary to the use of the object created.

Without consuming the time of the physiologist who is familiar with the form of the body and the laboratory processes of the stomach, bowel, peritoneum, omentum and all the parts interested in the production of pure arterial blood from crude material, we will start with the chyle that is deposited in the receptaculum chyli. This fluid is conducted through the thoracic duct to the veins where the union of the impure venous blood and the impure chyle takes place. It then passes on to the heart and thence to the lungs where the impurities are separated from the pure substances and are thrown off. After the process of refinement in the lungs the pure arterial blood returns to the heart to receive such qualifications as are necessary before it is passed into the arteries and conducted to its destination in the various parts of the body. I have no doubt whatever that when each organ receives its quota of blood from the arterial system, that organ by addition, subtraction and otherwise, prepares this fluid for its local use and passes it on to the nerve system for its cellular action previous to applying it as bone, muscle and tissue. The heart, the fountain of life, is the organ in the human body which imparts the attributes of life and knowledge to the blood so that it can proceed correctly with all its work.

I do not need to learn the form nor physical actions of the heart but I want to know what attributes of life are located in the heart between conception and manhood. We have no doubt of the powers of the mind and life to plan and build. We see the work of life as the voucher of what it can do. We know that life through the machinery of the body which it has made for all its uses, can manufacture and apply all substances in form to compose bone, muscle and other tissues. The important question at this time is, who or what power conducts the mental part of this work? Is life a substance? Is it a being above electricity, oxygen and other invisible substances, which is endowed with powers of mind to plan and use the forces of the elements in its work? If so, we have a reason why life never fails to produce the perfect in all its work.

DISEASES OF THE HEART.

Heart disease is never found without an impingement of the pneumogastric nerve at some point. Palpitation is an effect only, the result of an effort of the heart to force blood through capillaries to the venous system and back to the heart but which fails for lack of vital force. The lack of nerve force to empty the veins is the local cause of venous congestion, thus a rebound of blood at the heart. Still we have not found the cause of the failure of nerve force to empty the capillaries into the veins, thence to the heart nor can we until we examine the pneumogastric nerve and find the point on that nerve where force is cut off or weakened by some pressure on the nerve. As the pneumogastric nerve supplies both the heart and lung I am quite sure if the heart is weak or over-active that the cause will be found to be in the nerve supply of the lung, and the heart's extra effort is because the functioning of the lungs is imperfect. They fail to receive and return the blood normally. Thus the continuous effort of the heart increases in proportion to the venous congestion of the lungs which is one cause of palpitation of the heart.

At this point of our observation we reason that if the chest is occupied by congested lungs the blood is held back to give more room for the lungs to act. But as the heart fills anew after every stroke, and blood that is already in the artery cannot go either way, it becomes a stationary bumper. Then the heart makes a heroic effort to overcome the resistance caused by the blood that is piled up in the arterial tunnel and the local obstruction causes the heart to labor faster and faster with all its powers to drive the blood on and out of the artery and remove the obstruction to the normal passing of the blood from and to the heart.

So far we have only found effects and are not ready to treat our patient because we have not found the first cause that has led to the effects. We must hunt till we find the cause of the furious commotion of the heart and lungs or we will do the patient no good. We must know where to start or we shall fail. The heart must have rest or death will close the battle and we will be defeated because we have combated only the smoke of the enemy's artillery. Now we will start out with the search-light of reason and carefully explore the pneumogastric nerve and all its branches. If the branches of that nerve that supply the lungs are impinged upon or weakened at any point, the lungs cannot do perfect work in preparing blood by chemical action. Then we see that the lung fails to do its work, and the heart suffers as an effect of lung failure. The lungs have failed because the respiratory nerves have been disabled by pressure of spine, ribs or muscles and deranged in their functioning in the lungs. Thus we see that the heart gets in trouble after the lung fails and the lung fails after the respiratory branches of the pneumogastric nerves have been overcome by pressure, wounds or any other cause that would suspend their action.

What would cause fatty degeneration of the heart? Is congestion of the lung the cause of that soft and fatty appearance of the heart? Yes, the blood having stopped in and enlarged the lung and filled the thorax produces back pressure in the right side of the heart which causes stagnation of venous blood in the coronary veins and the heart becomes exhausted in its efforts to force blood into and out of the lungs while its nutrition is interfered with and softening and fatty degeneration of the heart muscle follow. All this trouble is the result of paralysis of the respiratory nerves. The same thing—paralysis of the lungs—would cause congestion of liver, spleen, kidney and all organs below the respiratory system.

HICCUP.

Definition of Singultus.—Hiccough or hiccup. A noise made by the sudden and involuntary contraction of the diaphragm, and the simultaneous contraction of the glottis arresting the air in the trachea; it is a symptom of many morbid conditions, but occurs frequently in persons otherwise in good health.

—Dunglison.

Etiology.—In all the cases of hiccups that I have examined during the last thirty-five years, I have found soreness on both sides and in front of the neck in the region of the pneumogastric and phrenic nerves. I have also found soreness on both sides of the spinous processes of the cervical and dorsal vertebrae as low down as the ninth. I have found much rigidity of the muscles in the regions named. I find the first rib on one side, sometimes on both, down and back and in between its own and the next process. I also find the clavicle on one or both sides dropped down from its articulation with the sternum, and the scapular end far back on the acromian process, and in some cases, cutting off or disturbing the intercostal blood and nerve supply as low as the diaphragm.

Treatment.—I carefully adjust all of the bones of the neck region including the clavicles and the hyoid bone; all of the dorsal vertebrae and the ribs. I carefully examine to see that each one is in its natural position. I want to give perfect freedom to the great splanchnic nerves from their origin clear on through the diaphragm to the solar plexus, because I think much of the trouble in hiccups comes from the obstruction that the great splanchnic meets as it passes through the diaphragm to the semilunar ganglion. I aim to give perfect freedom to that system of nerves. It must be freed as it passes through the diaphragm. The whole right side, every rib and vertebra clear on down to the sacrum should be carefully inspected to know they are in perfect line, because of the number of nerves that pass out in this region. I examine the lumbar region and if any variations of the bony processes are found, correct them and try to leave my patient, when he is not too far exhausted by some disease, free from the irritation which results in what is known as hiccups.

ABDOMINAL REGION

DIGESTION.

Definition.—The process by means of which alimentary substances, when introduced into the digestive canal, undergo different alterations. The object of it is to convert them into two parts: the one, a reparatory juice, destined to renew the perpetual waste occurring in the economy; the other, deprived of its nutritious properties, to be rejected from the body. This is affected by a series of organic actions differing according to the particular organization of the animal. In man they are eight in number—viz., prehension of food, mastication, insalivation, deglutition, action of the stomach, action of the small intestine (that of the bile, pancreatic juice, and intestinal secretion), action of the large intestine, expulsion of the faeces. Digestion is also a pharmaceutical operation which consists in treating certain solid substances with water, alcohol, or other menstruum, at a slightly elevated temperature, in a sand bath for example, or by leaving them exposed for some time to the sun.

—*Dunglison.*

Today we know about as little of the process of atomizing food as Adam and Eve did when they ate their first apples. We find fluids of different kinds in the stomach, bowel, pancreas, liver, omentum and peritoneum. We analyze them and find differences in the substances of each division. We name each fluid, talk of chemical action, call this process digestion and stop. We find that fluids are collected in a tank called the receptaculum chyli and from there they are conducted by way of the thoracic duct to the veins, the heart, thence to the lungs and here we drop the subject of digestion. We ask no questions of Edison, Morse or Franklin about the power of electricity to atomize food or to explode compounds while in the stomach. Perhaps an electrician would tell us that the heart is a dynamo, the brain is a storage battery, and the nerves are the wires that conduct the electricity to the stomach and bowels where it atomizes the food. Perhaps Edison would say the stomach and bowels are only vessels to hold the chemical compounds till electricity produces the act of combustion, and that electric combustion is all there is to digestion.

The body of man or beast shows to the electrician that absolutely perfect preparation has been provided for the generation, storing and application of electricity. By examining we see all acids and minerals necessary for vats and storage batteries. Then the heart is the engine to give motion to the electricity and the nerves are the wires for conducting it. The secretions of the alimentary canal are a part of the electrical apparatus. If the body is a machine then we can expect to find preparation for perfect work in all the parts.

I reason that when compounds are prepared in the stomach and bowels and are in a condition to receive the electricity from the nerves that terminate in the mucous membrane of the stomach and the rest of the alimentary canal, then Life as the engineer of the electric machine, touches the button, the heart begins, strikes and intermits and thus generates the electricity which is taken up by the nerve terminals in the blood vessels and carried to the storage battery by which it is delivered to the nerve terminals in the mucous membrane of the alimentary canal. From these nerve terminals there is a transfer of electricity to the food to be atomized and by the action of the electricity there is a separation of the molecules contained in the substances that are to be digested. From the heart as the center of force electricity carries on the process of delivering blood by way of the arteries and other fluids and gases by way of the excretories.

Digestion is the act of reduction; the process of reducing solids to fluids for nutrient purposes. I believe that electricity is the force and substance by which this result is obtained. Electricity as a force has no choice of what kind of substance it will tear asunder. It would just as soon spend its force on the wet as the dry; on the simple as the compound. If it approaches a simple substance, it will by its active force atomize that substance as well as another. It will not only atomize the substance of an explosive compound, but also prove its power of compatibility by combustion. On the subject of digestion, with the eye and mind of a critic, the eye of an engineer, the eye of a chemist, the eye of a practical electrical engineer who knows the action in all particulars of the perfectly constructed and wisely adjusted engine (which is found in the human body in which are the parts and complete engine) we see nothing but perfection in object and result—a most wonderful combination to plan for and use all physical forces, both explosive and cohesive, both mental and physical.

As I understand it this is the complete process of digestion, or the atomizing of substances by electricity. Another force is just as necessary to take up the atoms and apply them to the formation of bone, muscle fiber and so on. This force cannot be explosive but cohesive, and is known as magnetism. It comes to take the atoms in regular systematic order and adjust them according to form and place. You see in the first (electricity as a digestive force), the law of separation and destruction; in the latter (magnetism as a constructing force), the law of attraction and construction. By this process of reasoning we have some facts in place of theories to present to the explorer for truth, on the hitherto unknown process of digestion.

DYSPEPSIA.

Definition.—Indigestion difficulty of digestion. State of the stomach in which its functions are disturbed, without the presence of other diseases, or when, if other diseases be present, they are of but minor importance. Symptoms of dyspepsia are very various. Those affecting the stomach itself are loss of appetite, nausea, pain in the epigastrium or hypochondrium, heartburn, sense of fulness or weight in the stomach, acrid or fetid eructations, pyrosis, and sense of fluttering or sinking at the pit of the stomach. Sympathetic affections are of the most diversified character. Dyspepsia is generally functional, but when arising from disease of the stomach itself is, of course, serious. Dyspepsia may be of duodenal origin, duodenal or intestinal dyspepsia, and is generally accompanied with pain over that bowel some hours after food has been taken. As dyspepsia is usually dependent on irregularity of living, either in quantity or quality of the food taken, the most successful treatment is to put the patient on a diet easy of digestion; to combat the causes when such are apparent; and, by proper remedies and regimen, to strengthen the system in every practicable manner. It is often connected with inflammatory or subinflammatory condition of the mucous lining of the stomach. It may be attended with too great a secretion of the gastric acids, acid dyspepsia; but these sometimes appear to be too small in quantity, so as to constitute alkaline or neutral indigestion.

—*Dunglison.*

Etiology and Examination.—What organ of the whole abdomen is without a connecting branch between itself and the solar plexus? If the nerve and blood supply and the proper functioning of each organ of the abdomen are dependent upon the solar plexus, then when we have a dyspeptic for diagnosis and treatment we will go up to the origin of the great splanchnics in the spinal cord and come down through the diaphragm and semilunar ganglia to the solar plexus, searching for the trouble. Explore the spine in the region of the branching off of the splanchnic nerves which connect with terminals and supply the semilunar ganglia. If you find the fifth, sixth, seventh or eighth ribs of the right side are in malposition, you are on the right track and know why we have a diseased solar plexus. It is because of the failure of the semilunar ganglia to furnish to the solar plexus such supplies as it is the duty of these ganglia to furnish.

Should the food lie heavy on the stomach, with much flatulence, explore the left side of the spine and ribs beginning with the first and continuing to the ninth. You will find a failure of the solar plexus to prepare and deliver a sufficient quantity of alkaline substances to neutralize all over-plusses of acids, which results in lack of harmony in the processes of digestion. In all cases of indigestion you will find tenderness in the region of the solar plexus. You will also find imperfect functioning of the solar plexus.

Treatment.—Begin at the sacrum and bring the facets of the fifth lumbar forward until it articulates properly with the sacrum, then properly adjust each section of the lumbar spine. Continue your exploration from the twelfth dorsal up to the fifth ribs or higher on both sides. Adjust all variations. Then lay patient on right side and gently pull the stomach towards the left side in order to relieve the solar plexus from any ligation of nerve and blood supply by pressure of the stomach or bowels. Such pressure prevents free action of the nerve and blood supply and venous drainage of all organs of the abdomen. By this method the excretory system acts to renovate, and the secretory system acts to repair and strengthen all branches of the solar plexus necessary to healthy action. When this is established normal digestion results and all the symptoms common to dyspepsia will disappear.

DISEASES OF THE LIVER.

Etiology and Examination.—When a mechanic finds an abnormally large liver he begins to look for the shut-off or pressure that has stopped the blood from passing to and away from the liver. With the presence of impoverished venous blood, water, lymph or any other fluid that is not of vital importance to that organ he knows that he has temporary or permanent paralysis of the hepatic system, or of the nerves that act on the excretory system of that organ. He carefully examines the spine from the fifth to the ninth dorsal on the right side to see if the great splanchnic is oppressed or its normal action suspended by ribs thrown from their normal articulation. He explores carefully the fifth, sixth, seventh and eighth ribs on the left side because he wants a good healthy action of the spleen and pancreas, the diaphragm and all nerves going to or from the solar plexus. Then he continues his exploration on the upper dorsal to ascertain if there is any lateral deviation of the upper eight dorsal vertebra or ribs, because if he is a mechanic who knows his business, he finds the cause of inhibition and paralysis of the hepatic branches of the solar plexus by this examination. When exploring the upper dorsal to find if there is any lateral, anterior or posterior curvature of the spine in this region, he expects to find the cause that he knows has produced this condition of the liver, which is due to local paralysis of the nerves that are responsible for its normal action.

Treatment.—After the description just given I think the operator is just about ready to proceed to adjust the spine from the occiput to the sacrum after the manner given in other chapters on spine and rib adjustment.

If the upper dorsal presents an imperfect alignment of the spinous processes (and often when the spinous processes are all in a straight line), on careful examination we may find lateral curvature with convex bulging to the right or to the left, from the second to the eighth dorsal. A good method of correcting such is to hook your fingers strongly on the opposite side of the spinous processes and in the concavity of the curvature, then push the neck, not the head but the *neck* towards that concavity. Then I place my upper hand on the back of the neck and bend the neck forward and down with a rotary motion. We should adjust all ribs carefully in this region, and never treat such cases more than once or twice a week for fear of unnecessary soreness. As to diet and exercise let the patient use his own judgment. This is not at all important. I could make a list of a large number of diseases or effects—called diseases of the liver—which would be of very little use to a mechanic who is exploring the body to find the cause or causes that produce such effects. His question is this, "where is the friction that is responsible for the trouble?" He will not be satisfied until he knows he has explored and corrected all nerve and blood supply, and the natural drainage of that organ.

I think in this day and generation, if you open and peruse all medical books you will find seventy-five per cent of the work has been devoted to describing and naming effects, in place of finding the cause of the disease. I think it is high time that we take our eyes off the smoke, and hunt until we find the fire that produces the effect. It is not wisdom to spend any more time in analyzing and classifying the different chemical substances found in the smoke. I think it would be greater wisdom, if we wish to change the smoke, or effect, to find the furnace before we expect to control the cause that produces the various kinds of smoke which are effects only.

GALL-STONES.

Definition.—A concretion of cholesterin or inspissated bile formed in the gall-bladder or one of the bile-ducts; see Calculi, biliary.

Biliary Calculi.—Biliary concretions, gall-stones, some being nothing more than secretion of bile thickened; the greater part are composed of cholesterin, with some coloring matter of bile; biliary calculi are most frequently found in the gall bladder, cystic calculi; at other times in the substance of the liver, in branches of the ductus hepaticus, hepatic calculi; or in the ductus communis choledochus, hepatocystic calculi.

—*Dunglison.*

Under definition of *Calculi*, Dunglison says, "Their solution is generally impossible; nature must remove them by spontaneous expulsion, or, failing this, extraction by surgical measures is the only practicable way of getting rid of them."

We have given you above Dunglison's definitions which give all such cases but little hope of relief short of a surgical operation which, according to my observation, is of very little if any benefit. I will give the student the benefit of my experience and tell him of my success in cause-hunting for gall-stones and in giving relief from the suffering which they cause. I have had a great many well-defined cases of gall-stones which I have treated successfully, and my patients got well without the use of the knife or any sort of drug. I will give you the history of a few of these cases.

About twelve years ago Judge Springer of the United States Court of the State of Arkansas brought his wife to me for treatment. She was suffering greatly. There was great misery in the right side, in the region of the gall-duct. When I was called to her she was in an unconscious state, or a spasmodic condition. I made an examination and found a large lump just a little above and to the right of the umbilicus, which I diagnosed at once as a gall-stone. Upon this diagnosis I proceeded to treat my patient, adjusting the spine and lower ribs and finishing my work by pressing the stone gently in the direction of the stomach. Soon the lump gave way and disappeared. Within an hour from the time I pressed the gall-stone out of the gall-duct she regained consciousness and she never experienced any further trouble with gall-stones. The next day she passed a gall-stone as large as a small walnut, after which she passed a few about the size of hazelnuts. She lived about eight years after this attack, with perfect comfort as far as gall-stones were concerned.

Some ten or twelve years ago a Mr. Dufrey of Schuyler County, Mo., came to me suffering with what the medical doctors called biliary colic. He was insane from the misery he was suffering. While in that condition he struck the wife of Dr. Patterson a blow on her breast with such force as to break loose two or three ribs from the sternum. I had several stout men take hold of him, throw him down on the ground and hold him until I could search for gall-stones, which I soon discovered to be in the gall-duct. I treated him and then pushed the stones on, and out of the gall-duct, giving instantaneous relief both to body and mind. The next day he passed off and brought to me a gall-stone about the size of a pigeon's egg with several smaller ones. After this he passed many, and came to me with the report that he had washed the fecal matter and found and counted over one hundred small stones.

Another case was that of Mrs. Hunt of Minneapolis who came to me about fifteen years ago stating that she was then suffering excruciating pains in her right side, between her liver and stomach, and that the medical doctor called it biliary colic. This patient was a very fleshy woman, notwithstanding which I could feel that the gall-duct was fully as large as my thumb. I proceeded the first thing to push what I considered to be the stones out of the gall-duct giving her immediate relief. I have known this patient ever since and she tells me that she never has had any return of what the doctors called biliary colic.

Now that I have given you the history of these cases I will say that I have examined and treated successfully many other patients suffering with gall-stones, during the many years in which I have practiced the principles of osteopathy as a remedy for the cure of this agonizing disease.

Etiology.—In my opinion gall-stones are the result of temporary paralysis of the splanchnic nerve system which I have found compressed by the malposition of the fifth, sixth, seventh or eighth ribs on either or both sides. I have never found a case of gall-stones where there was perfect rib articulation with the transverse processes of the fifth, sixth, seventh and eighth vertebrae.

I think this paralysis produces a failure of the liver, spleen and pancreas to carry out their functions to such a degree as to prevent the liver from excreting sufficient oily matter to supply the gall-bladder with oil enough to keep the chalk from forming gall-stones. I have here given you my opinion based upon many years successful work in treating such diseases. I have given you a lengthy description in order that I may give you a short, comprehensive and reliable method of successful treatment.

Treatment.—When I am called to a patient suffering with such miseries in the right side in the region of the gall-bladder, I lay my patient on his back, flex and bring the knees up far enough to slack the abdominal muscles in order that I may explore in the region of the gall-duct for any foreign substance. I will say to the operator that this is no place for gouging with the points of the fingers. If you ever intend to be useful by working in this region with your fingers lay them flat. While you are sitting on the left side of your patient, bring your elbow up towards the patient's right shoulder, lay your hand easily on the side of your patient, letting your fingers extend about three inches below the umbilicus. Now remember what I tell you, none of your gouging, but feel easily in the region of the gall-duct. Then with your right little finger back of the lump push it from the gall-duct to the left slowly and easily, holding the little finger firmly to the place. Then bring the next finger alongside of the little finger and firmly hold it to place. Then the middle finger, holding it firmly a while. Then bring the index finger to bear firmly but gently behind the lump. Each finger in turn reinforcing the first. Be patient, move slowly and give the gall-duct time to dilate. About this time the lump will disappear, as it enters the intestine. Now you have given relief which always follows delivery of the gall-stones. Before you leave your patient carefully adjust the vertebrae of the dorsal and lumbar regions, then turn him on his right side and carefully adjust all the ribs of the left side, because you want no intercostal blood or nerve stagnation. Now have your patient turn on the left side, while you stand in front of him and carefully adjust all of the ribs of his right side to their natural articulation. Give this treatment about twice each week. I have generally kept patients suffering with gall-stones or biliary colic under my observation for two or three months.

CONSTIPATION.

Definition.—Costiveness, fecal retention, alvine obstruction, stopping or stoppage of the bowels; state of the bowels in which the evacuations do not take place as frequently as usual, or are inordinately hard and expelled with difficulty, owing to diminished action of the muscular coat of the intestines or to diminished secretion from the mucous membrane, or to both. The exciting and predisponent causes must be inquired into and obviated to render the cure permanent. A distinction is sometimes made between constipation (infrequency of stool) and costiveness (dryness and hard ness of the faeces).

—Dunglison.

Etiology.—Here we have the popular definition of constipation as given by Dunglison, which is about all the light that any author throws on this subject before the plan of medication begins. This amounts to very little to an osteopath who well knows the effects of constipation, such as hard feces which are very difficult to expel from the bowels, and he mentally asks the question, what is wrong with the machine? If he understands his anatomy and physiology he goes to the brain, the spinal cord, the solar plexus and all the nerves which supply the structures of the abdomen, as well as to the arterial supply, the venous drainage, the lymphatic system and the biliary system, asking as he goes, where is the shut-off which interferes with the normal supply of the fluids of the body without which a normal action of the bowels cannot be expected?

He reasons that if there is headache, hysteria, enlarged uterus, kidney trouble, either too much or too little urine, he must begin his work at the atlas and free up both nerve and blood supply. He reasons further that it is impossible to have perfect order in any organ or structure of the body when there is a constriction at the point where the nerve supply leaves the head to enter the spinal column, the main route over which the nerves pass and from which they branch off for special and general purposes. He knows that from about the fifth to the eighth dorsal the great splanchnic branches off, passes to the solar plexus and arrives at the semilunar ganglion. With this knowledge he concludes what has caused this condition. On this conclusion he proceeds to correct the whole spinal system and its branches and free it from every obstruction to normal nerve action.

He knows that the constricting cause is between the occiput and the coccyx. He knows that there is a shortage of the lymphatic fluids that should constantly keep the bowels or the fecal matter in a soft condition. Thus can be seen the importance of venous liberty. He knows that from the abdominal aorta comes the blood supply to the intestines, colon and the kidneys, and also that the aorta goes to the pelvis and there breaks up into many branches supplying the bladder, the uterus and so on. Each organ receives its arterial blood, does its work, and tries to deliver the venous blood, and will do so normally when nothing interferes. But when the pelvis is crowded and impacted with bowel, uterus, bladder, fecal matter or any foreign growths he must get a free return of the venous blood with a normal action of the lymphatics, in order that they may throw off the watery fluids to supply the intestines. He can expect normal action of bowel to appear very soon after the drawing up of the viscera from out its impacted condition in the pelvic cavity.

Treatment.—In treating constipation which has become anything like chronic, I always begin with the atlas. I want to know about any variation in the articulation of the atlas with the head, and also to know that I can detect it when it does exist. I make it my object to explore for, to detect and correct any and all abnormalities of this articulation. I generally find the neck humped up, dropped in or pushing out at one side or the other.

Starting at the atlas I proceed to go over every bone in the neck and adjust each one to the normal because without a normal spinal cord from origin to destination we can not expect good results. As the spinal cord goes on farther than the neck we must continue our search down the spine stopping to adjust both clavicles and the scapulae, leaving them in a normal position. Continuing on to the region between the fourth and the twelfth dorsal we examine very carefully here both vertebrae and ribs, adjusting and testing each separately, in order to make sure that the splanchnic nerves as well as the blood vessels in this region are unobstructed.

Then the lumbar vertebrae are to be adjusted carefully. In doing this one method is to have your patient get on his knees on the floor. Let the breast be supported by a stool about fourteen inches high so that it will drop the body downward a little, then coming up behind the patient take his thighs between your knees firmly and rotate the patient with your knees with a twisting motion, a little to right and then to the left keeping your hands or thumbs at each vertebra till you have them in perfect articulation from the sacrum to the twelfth dorsal. This twisting, rotating motion loosens all the facets of the lumbar vertebrae. While my patient is in this position I reach underneath his abdomen with both hands and gently draw the contents of both abdomen and pelvis up and forward towards the navel which will relieve an impacted pelvis. This I do with flat hands, and I mean *flat hands*. Keep the points of your fingers out of all abdomens because if you do not you will bruise a kidney, a ureter, a spleen, the peritoneum, the omentum or the liver all of which are liable to injury by rough handling.

In severe cases I would advise that the bowel be filled with thin flour gruel every few days in order that the colon can have nourishment and also that a separation of the dry fecal matter from the walls of the bowel can take place. Teach your patient how to take the knee-chest position and gently draw the contents of the pelvis and lower abdomen up, and direct him to do it every night at bed time. Give your constipated patients the plain ordinary diet with plenty of water to drink. In treating after this manner I have had good success with all cases except those of a purely surgical type. In a large per cent of so-called cases of appendicitis, by following this treatment you will have no use for the knife.

DIARRHEA.

Definition.—Looseness of the bowels; purging; scouring. Disease characterized by frequent liquid alvine evacuations, and generally owing to inflammation or to irritation of the mucous membrane of the intestines. It is often caused by errors in regimen, the use of food noxious by its quality and quantity.

—Dunglison.

Etiology.—I have given you above my philosophy and method of treatment in cases of constipation, which has restored the bowels to their normal action in the majority of cases that I have treated, thereby gaining very satisfactory results and finding that Nature when unobstructed can do such work as is required of each organ. The intestines are not excepted from Nature's unerring laws.

In treating constipation I began with the atlas because I could find somewhere between the occiput and the coccyx, obstructive causes that would prohibit the production and the delivery of the natural lubricating fluids to the large and small intestines. I draw your attention here to the treatment of constipation, beginning at the head and ending at the coccyx, because of the need of a reversal of this method in a successful treatment of diarrhea, dysentery and bloody flux which is a watery, slimy or bloody alvine discharge due to and resulting from obstruction and irritation in the lumbar region, or in some cases in the dorsal up as high as the fourth.

Throughout this region I explore very thoroughly because no irritative, obstructive condition of the nerves can be tolerated with any hope of ease, comfort or normal action of the lower bowels. Among other causes giving rise to such nerve irritation are to be noted the eating of unripe fruits, the drinking of impure water; the use of fermented milk, ice cream, or other foods which are in a decomposing state; too large a secretion of bile; sudden atmospheric changes; also poisonous gases rising from the earth, ground or swamps at a season when days are hot, nights are cold or there is much dampness. Such gases on uniting with the venous blood and fluids that are sent to the lungs to go through the process of producing pure arterial blood have a poisonous effect. There is a failure in the perfection of arterial blood to its highest degree of vitality before it is sent forth to do its duty, and arterial blood below the average is always followed by a failure in the abdominal viscera to retain its normal condition; then we may expect such irritations as result in the bowels losing their power to secrete nutrition, and instead, becoming excretory in the highest degree and throwing off their contents in fluid form.

Treatment.—I will now give you one of many methods that have proved effective in many cases of diarrhea which I have been called upon to treat. When my patient is a stout man I generally stand him in a doorway and place his breast and abdomen against the jamb of the door. I then stand behind him and place my knee on the upper part of the sacrum so as to bring the spinous process of the fifth lumbar against my knee and give fairly strong pressure. By taking hold of his shoulders I bring his back firmly towards my knee with the object of raising the fifth lumbar from the sacrum. Then swing him to the right and left a few times so as to open out and loosen up all of the lumbar articulations with a view of freeing the whole nervous system of the lower spine from any impingement whatever. Now I turn my patient so that he will face me with his back against the door-jamb. I take him by both shoulders, and push them backwards to secure good blood circulation of the upper dorsal region. Now seat the patient on a stool, stand in front of him and have him place both his arms over your shoulders. Place your arms around his body with your hands each side of the twelfth dorsal vertebra, the place of beginning of this part of the treatment. I carefully examine and adjust every dorsal vertebra and also the ribs which articulate with them. With my hands each side of the spine I gently but firmly draw the patient towards me and know that freedom is given the blood and nerve supply in this region. The clavicles and the cervical vertebrae now receive careful attention and adjustment, not leaving my patient until I have perfect articulation from the sacrum to the occiput. When there is much headache I generally inhibit the occipital nerves in the back part of the neck.

I give such treatments two or three times the first day provided my first treatment has failed to give perfect ease. I have my patient lie down and rest after the treatment and when there is much griping and suffering, after an hour or so, I have the lower bowel filled with a thin flour gruel, not starch, the formula for which I have given you. This I do because of the contact of the raw and unprotected surfaces of the bowel. Then let the patient while resting or sleeping lie mostly on the right side because when in that position there is less tendency for the bowel to become impacted in the pelvis. Keep all washes and douches out of the bowel except this nutritious gruel.

For a few days feed the patient on light, easily digestible food. I never allow my patient to eat such things as pickles or green fruit. Have the patient in a comfortable room and away from the glaring light and heat of the sun. I want to caution you against severe and rough treatments. When my patient is a woman, or a man too ill to get up, I treat them in their bed while they lie either on their face or side, and go over the work as I have outlined, only very gently and carefully and without any violence.

Babes and children up to the age of five or six I generally take up in my lap as I sit in a chair and have them throw their arms over my shoulders. Then I begin at the fifth lumbar and adjust from the sacrum to the occiput remembering that I am handling a child and knowing well that it requires but little force to adjust and loosen up the entire spine. In these little ones, I generally find the abdomen very cold and the entire spine and the head very hot. Both these conditions soon disappear after the adjustment of the spine and ribs.

DYSENTERY.

Definition.—Bloody flux; flux. Inflammation of the mucous membrane of the large intestine, the chief symptoms of which are fever, more or less inflammatory, with frequent mucous or bloody evacuations violent tormina, and tenesmus. When the evacuations do not contain blood it has been called simple dysentery. The seat of the disease is generally in the colon and rectum; it occurs particularly during the summer and autumnal months, and in hot climates more than in cold; frequently also in camps and prisons, from impure air and imperfect nourishment, and is often epidemic. Sporadic cases of dysentery are generally easily managed, but when epidemic it often exhibits great malignancy.

—Dunglison.

Symptoms.—Bilious fever or dysentery generally be gins with running off of the bowels, sick stomach, with chilliness of the whole body alternating with fever, and the suffering extends from the brain to the lower extremity of the spine. Nausea is one of the first symptoms, and is soon followed by a watery and loose discharge from the bowels which continues for a few hours or a number of days and is accompanied by a griping and bearing down of the lower bowel. In many cases blood passes off with the fecal discharges. There is generally a continual fever of the head and spine with a cold abdomen. This condition is generally known as summer complaint, dysentery or flux.

Etiology.—Now you have your patient, what will you do with him? How will you proceed to ascertain what is the cause of this trouble? We reason that the spine has been exposed to the sun and the body has been exercised sufficiently to irritate the whole spinal column with its nerves and their branches, from the brain to the coccyx. You ask what effect this would have. Irritation of the spinal cord, and all the nerves to the bowels in particular, will produce contracture of the muscles of the spine strong enough to shut off the nerves of the excretory system. Then the urine fails to pass off and carry away fluids and substances that are fermenting in the excretory ducts, and the bowel fails to throw off the substances fermenting in its lining membrane. Now you have a congested condition, a stopping and retention of the contents and substances of the bowels. This is accompanied by bloody discharges. By the fluids being retained you have inflammation, fermentation and sloughing off of the mucous membrane. In these summer affections just spoken of you will find a very hot feverish condition extending the whole length of the spine from the occiput to the coccyx. The spine is hot because of fermentation which is Nature's method of reducing these substances into a gaseous or fluid condition so they may pass off through the excretories more easily when the nerves of the excretory system are freed from the irritation that would produce contracture.

Prognosis.—In your expectations or prognosis you must make allowance for the health and the general condition of the system of your patient when attacked. If these summer complaints should attack with great severity a person who has been suffering from pulmonary or abdominal diseases the case is far less hopeful than if the patient were strong and robust at the time the disease of the bowels appeared.

Treatment.—You will find in your treatment of flux that the third, fourth and fifth lumbar vertebrae are far back on the sacrum. This posterior condition often extends as high up as the tenth dorsal and your work is to adjust the articulations from the tenth dorsal to the fifth lumbar and take off all irritation. By this you prepare the lower system for renovation through the excretories. By doing this the osteopath gets the desired results without recourse to opiates, drugs or enemata which are wholly unnecessary.

As soon as you have the spine adjusted to the truly normal, misery gives place to ease in the lower bowel. Carefully journey up with your hands to the eighth, seventh, sixth and fifth ribs. See that no rib has left its normal position on its transverse process. Then proceed with the fourth, third, second and first ribs and know that they and the upper dorsal vertebrae are all in line because the nervous system in this region supplies the lungs with a class of nutrient fluid that causes them to generate water, which is soon taken up by the secretions of the lungs and passed out of the body through the excretory system. By close observation you will find the variations and be rewarded by good results if your patient has called on you in anything like reasonable time.

Your work is to see that the spinal nerves are in such a condition that they can do normal work. Take all irritating pressures off the nerve system of the whole spine. In short, have a good correct spine and you may expect good results for your patient and satisfaction to yourself as an operator. For thirty years I have demonstrated that bowel complaints were very submissive to a corrected spine. It is not necessary for you to annoy the bowels by pulling, hauling or rubbing, but gently lift them from the pelvis while your patient is in the knee-chest position. Outside of that you are liable to do much mischief and increase the ravages of the inflammation. If the patient is very weak inject some warm gruel into the lower bowel.

I have found in all of my practice, and have been surprised to know, that at roll call Nature always answered "present" with her remedies. By adjusting the spine from the sacrum to the occiput you have set at liberty the nerves that control the bowels from the rectum up the full extent of the descending, transverse and ascending colon, down to the cecum, ileocecal valve, intestine and back to its union with the stomach, the stomach itself and up the whole extent of the esophagus. Thus you are admonished by that condition to adjust every vertebra and know that its facets articulate with those of its fellow and that every facet and rib is in its normal position. In adjusting the Spine and all of its articulations with the ribs and all other parts a demand is made for your skill. Here is your field of labor in summer complaints and all diseases pertaining to the esophagus, stomach, small and large intestine to its terminal.

Now I have given the osteopath the idea upon which to work. He or she who knows the framework will know what they must do and by very little skill will succeed in adjusting every part to the normal. I want to say once and for all that in every case of dysentery, constipation or stagnation of the bowels in a person who is otherwise normal, this condition is an effect of an abnormal spine. By abnormal spine I mean a variation of one section of the spine with another, or the ribs being thrown off the transverse processes and obstructing the intercostal supply of the vein, nerve and artery. It matters not what name you call it, here is your mystery. Govern yourself accordingly. I have found this method of procedure to be perfectly satisfactory in all cases from infancy to old age.

When your patient is a child you will find that its back will be hot the entire length of the spine and its belly cold as clay from its nipples to the pubis. Its buttocks are also cold. A very good way to treat the child is to put its breast to your breast, begin with your hands at the sacrum and gently work up and adjust its spine. Its back will get cool and a pleasant warm perspiration will break out and it will go to sleep. One says, "what will you feed it"? Hand it back to its mother and tell her to give it some fried breakfast bacon. This will pass through the stomach to the lower bowels and soothe by oiling the entire canal, the ileocecal valve and from there to the lower part of the rectum. Diet cuts but little figure with me. The usual diet of the home habit is best. I will say in conclusion use good common sense. If you have a case of bloody flux or anything of the kind give such a diet as is easily digested, keeping nuts and fresh fruits out of the way. Fresh buttermilk is good, ordinary bread has always been acceptable, but any mother should know enough to keep trash away from her child at such times.

APPENDICITIS.

Definition.—Inflammation of the vermiform appendix of the caecum.

Chronic Appendicitis.—Long-continued, low-grade inflammation of the vermiform appendix, interrupted from time to time by acute exacerbations; relapsing or recurrent appendicitis.

Appendicitis Obliterans.—Form of chronic appendicitis in which there is a progressive obliteration of the lumen of the appendix from fibrous new growth, contraction, or plastic peritonitis.

—*Dunglison.*

Etiology.—I have been consulted a great many times about appendicitis. I have had a considerable number of patients come to me with the report that their home physician had diagnosed their case as appendicitis and that there was no hope for a cure short of the use of the knife. Notwithstanding the fact that the medical fraternity had declared such cases to be appendicitis with the possibility and probability that the appendix was filled with seeds or some other foreign bodies I proceeded to treat according to the principles of our science and according to my conclusions, namely, that the soreness and irritation in the region of the ileocecal valve was caused by the structures here being pushed far down into the pelvis so that the cecum could not pass the fecal matter from the ileum to the colon. For over thirty years I have treated such cases successfully, basing my work you this philosophy. I have not made use of the knife in a single case nor had the loss of a patient.

Treatment.—I place my patient in the knee-chest position. Then lay my hands flat on the lower part of the abdomen and with a gentle pressure I draw the bowel, cecum and all of the structures in this region upward toward the diaphragm. I gently draw or press the entire contents of the lower abdomen up and out of the impacted condition they were in in the pelvis. While my patient is in the knee-chest position I proceed to adjust the entire spinal column after the manner which I have given you. Beginning with the coccyx and the sacrum adjust most carefully every articulation of vertebra with vertebra, and also with the ribs. Make sure that you free up both the nerve and blood supply to the region here affected. I want to emphasize that you should never use a knife with the hope that you can get more money than you could by good thorough osteopathic work.

I will give a case or two of so-called appendicitis. Judge Richards of Eudora, Kansas, wrote me that he had a son suffering with appendicitis; that a council of doctors had been called and that their decision was that his son must be operated on immediately in order to save his life. The Judge wanted to know if I could save his son from the knife and asked an answer by telegram. My answer was, yes. Inside of twelve hours he and his son were at my office in Kirksville, Mo. I proceeded immediately to relieve an impacted pelvis and to treat him according to osteopathic principles. Ease followed and two days later they went home to Kansas. This was twelve years ago and he has had no trouble of this kind since.

About nine years ago Dr. Hook while a student in my school was suffering excruciating pain low down in his right side. The wisest council of the town was given that the knife must be used inside of twelve hours or death must result. When I heard this decision I concluded I would go and see this patient myself. I found an impacted pelvis and a very sore cecum. Whether or not the appendix was inflamed was not the question. I treated this student, relieved the impacted pelvis, as well as the sore cecum, and in two days he was back in his place in school. He has never since had any symptoms of the disease.

I haven't the space to give you the history of hundreds of others whom I have treated for such suffering, during the last thirty-five years. I want to say to you, and to emphasize it, I think thousands of people are now in their graves because of the lack of mechanical skill in the doctor who has had charge of such cases.

TAPEWORM.

Definition.—A parasitic intestinal cestode worm, or species, of a flattened, tape-like form, and composed of separate joints. Those infesting man are principally of the genera Taenia and Bothriocephalus. The ova of tapeworms are taken into the alimentary canal of the host, whence they make their way into the tissues, where they form small cyst-like masses, called scolices or cysticerci.

When the flesh of the original host is eaten the scolices develop within the alimentary canal of the new host into a strobilus, or adult tapeworm, which consists of a head, neck, and a various (often very great) number of oblong joints, or segments, called proglottides, each of which is hermaphroditic and produces ova.

—Dorland.

As the osteopath may occasionally in his practice be consulted for the removal of a tapeworm, which is only known to be such by one or many joints passing away at stool, I think it would be well enough for me to give a short report of my treatment for tapeworm and of its success.

In the first place I will not take up time with historical theories as to how the tapeworm becomes an occupant of the human body. My object is to get them out of the body without the use of dangerous poisons whose after effects are as bad, or worse, than the tapeworm. I am of the opinion that with a healthy liver and a normal supply of healthy gall to the bowels the tapeworm will become sick, let loose all its hold and pass off with the fecal matter. While I have not had a very great number of such cases, I have succeeded in passing off the tapeworm, body and head.

I will tell the reader of my first case, which was in the southern part of Missouri. I remember that it was in 1888 at Nevada, Missouri. A homeopathic physician came in with a lady patient who was suffering from tapeworm, so he claimed. I asked how he knew she had a tapeworm. He said, "Because I have seen a number of joints that passed out with the fecal matter." He asked the question, "What can the 'bone doctor' do for tapeworm"? Knowing the origin, course and termination of the great splanchnic, I adjusted the spine and ribs in this region with the object of having the solar plexus nourished by the semilunar ganglia, then the solar plexus could reach and nourish the liver, and prepare it to generate and deliver gall to the bowels, which would sicken the tapeworm and drive it down and out. The next morning at ten o'clock the doctor and patient returned with the report that she had passed a tapeworm, body and head, and that it was twenty-seven feet long.

In another case, a man came to me to be treated for epilepsy. He said about three spasms or epileptic fits a month were the average. I examined him and found the upper ribs and dorsal vertebrae as low down as the ninth on the right side bulged out, and in a very abnormal condition at their articulations. I proceeded to adjust them with the hope that I had found the cause of epilepsy in his case. I treated him twice a week. During the second week I chanced to follow him to an outhouse and while there I noticed a white substance in bulk nearly a quart. I found that it was a pile of dead tapeworms about as large as my two fists; and that was the last of his convulsions. I give the two cases to encourage the osteopath to turn on the gall quickly and plenty of it when treating a case of fits or of tapeworm. Follow the great splanchnic, feed the solar plexus and the work is done.

DISEASES OF THE KIDNEYS.

The office of the kidney, or the duty to be performed by the kidney, is to collect and pass on through the bladder all substances entering into the composition of urine. The kidney will do all the services incumbent upon it just as long as there is no abnormality present. When an abnormality appears then the doctor's counsel, advice and treatment are sought. He prescribes what he calls kidney medicines or remedies, with the hope that normality will follow a use of such drugs. But in the course of time his patient reports no improvement, and in addition to the scanty or increased flow of urine there is blood and pus passed from the bladder with it. He stops the use of the medicines which he has prescribed without satisfactory results. He consults all the authors obtainable, finds another prescription for the kidneys that has done wonders in Scotland, England, Germany, France, Italy, North or South America. He sends off for this great kidney remedy. It arrives. His patient takes much or little according to the doctor's written prescription. A few weeks or months later he calls on the doctor, ghostly and pale in appearance, and notifies him that he grows weaker; his appetite is gone; some fever, and great suffering in the lower dorsal and lumbar regions. Counsel is called. Diagnosis: stone in the bladder, renal calculi. An operation is performed. No calculus is found either in the kidneys or bladder; the urine stops; blood poison follows the operation. Prostration and death in a few days. When the funeral is over and the doctor's bill is paid the story ends.

Etiology.—The same board is handed out for the next one to travel, from a dislocated back to the graveyard, and this has been and is today the procedure of the medical doctor in the treatment of kidney diseases. The osteopath looks at the framework of the spine, adjusts all variations that have followed strains, falls from horseback or down cellars, and partially or completely dislocated the ribs, lower dorsal or lumbar vertebrae to the degree of producing kidney diseases. The osteopath—not one with a diploma although without mechanical skill, but the osteopath who is a mechanic and knows his business—looks for causes, removes them, and cures his patient, provided the patient comes to him in reasonable time and is not eaten up with drugs, or inflammation following mechanical injuries to the spine.

Examination and Treatment.—For exploration place the patient at full length on the table, face down. With hands and head come down that spine as a fault finder and if you know your business as a mechanic you will find spinal variations between the eighth dorsal and the fifth lumbar. You are sure to find one or more of the ribs or vertebrae between the eighth dorsal and sacrum on a strain, twisted or partially dislocated. Then carefully explore as a critic the sacrum and coccyx, and adjust all variations you may find. My object in beginning at the eighth dorsal and coming down to the coccyx is to find and remove every cause that would hinder the kidney from receiving its full supply of arterial blood from the aorta at the point where the renal artery branches out for that organ. We should give the kidney a full quantity of blood because of the great quantity required by it.

Remember that you are expected to be very careful to leave the spine and ribs below the eighth in line so that the venous blood shall not be disturbed by any irritation that would produce contraction of the venous system before that blood arrives at the heart. We should make it a business to seek to know the cause and remove it. As to nourishment, I think the adult patient knows what and how much to eat, and when to quit. I think my advice is more needed on his back than at the table. I cannot afford to waste much time on dietetics. At an early day and as far back as I can recollect, honey has had a very popular place with the pioneers as a food when suffering in the back, or with kidney disease. The result has generally been very satisfactory. The more honey the patient would eat the sooner the spine and kidneys would get better. In all kidney diseases honey is very palatable as a diet. The quantity was limited by the appetite for the honey.

ABDOMINAL AND OTHER TUMORS.

Definition.—1. Swelling; morbid enlargement. 2. A neoplasm. A mass of new tissue which persists and grows independently of its surrounding structures, and which has no physiologic use. Tumors are innocent or malignant. Malignant tumors tend to infiltrate the tissues; innocent tumors push the tissues aside, and are usually encapsuled; many malignant tumors tend to produce secondary growths in adjacent glands, and are disseminated throughout the body; they affect the general health, and usually, when removed, tend to recur. There are many theories regarding the origin of tumors. The inclusion theory holds that tumors are developed from embryonic cells which were produced in greater numbers than the fetus required, and remain gathered in a certain point until stimulated to growth and development by physiologic activity of the part or the application of irritation. Some tumors are believed to be hereditary. Irritation and injury are thought by many to be the active agents in originating tumors. Physiologic activity aids the development of some forms, and physiologic decline of others.

—Dorland.

General Discussion.—Tumors are fatty, gristly or watery lumps, wads, or abnormal growths and accumulations. It is an abnormally big something inside of the skin, or of the body. Whether it is on the head, neck, chest, abdomen, legs, arms or skin it is an effect only of some cause. All things are produced by cause, so to treat simply effects in tumors is unwise. We may remove tumors with knife or drug, but others are very likely to appear unless we remove the cause. Thus osteopathy seeks to cure, not to waste flesh, blood or life, either by the knife or chloroform. The osteopath should labor to reduce the tumor without the knife. His remedy is normal nerve action and pure blood, and when the obstructing cause is removed in anything like reasonable time tumors will begin to disappear.

When this subject is brought before the mechanic's eye he takes a look, makes a mental note of the size, name, location and appearance of all unnatural growths found in the human body and gives special attention to the

156

one under consideration. By the marks of discrimination one is called malignant, another benign, another cancer, another fibroid, another cystic tumor, and so forth.

The anatomical physiologist in council would reason as a preserver of life, and would say to the surgeon: "We will be satisfied with nothing from nor tolerate any interference by the knife of any one who cannot give a demonstrable reason why this abnormal growth cannot be reduced without the knife. What important nerve of vaso-constriction or vaso-dilation has been prohibited from executing its work of normal construction and renovation to normal health?"

If the engineer approached the human body under the penalty of pain and death for spilling a single drop of blood or removing an atom of flesh if he failed to show and demonstrate the absolute cause that has produced this abnormally constructed thing or tumor; and if he knew that the penalty for a hasty conclusion and malpractice were death, he would become an earnest seeker for truth and a safe man to explore the abdomen to find and demonstrate the cause of cancers or tumefactions. The order under which he explores should demand wisdom and honesty and death should be the penalty if he fails to demonstrate the cause of such abnormal growths. Thus saith the Czar of the government under which this mechanic labors, and there is no appeal from the edict. As Christ did so shall he work without money or price.

If such were the law of our land it would soon abolish speculative murder, delay hundreds of thousands of funerals and save millions of yards of mourning crape which otherwise will be hung at the doors in almost every city and village. I want to insist that the time is fully ripe for legislative interference to stop the unwarranted use of the knife. I want to emphasize with vehemence that the hasty surgeon who can not demonstrate that he knows and has found the cause producing such a malady, but who wastes human life simply for the dollar that he can distort from the unfortunate sufferer or his friends by pretending to know the cause and by using the knife of death, should hang. Send a few such to the gallows or to the State prison for life for murder and this world will soon have surgery take its merited place. Give the surgeon of merit a reasonable reward fixed by law for his services, then we will have honest dealing with human life, and not before.

It is horrifying to think that we are living in a day and generation that sees nothing sacred in human life. I think it is time for legislation and legal interference to take command and regulate our system of surgery.

Following this prelude we can say something that will assist the osteopath in leaving the old rut of antiquated customs and in learning to hunt for and know the cause or causes producing tumors of the head, neck, thorax, mammary glands and all organs and limbs of the human body. I care nothing for analyzing the fluids of the body which are perverted from the normal. The question is what is the cause? How are we to know our conclusion is true? How can we demonstrate that what we say is a truth? Point it out before we proceed. We should give very careful attention to the blood supply of the abdomen and its organs, with its accompanying nerve forces, until we know the cause producing any abnormal effect. You should study until you can do this with credit, then proceed. If any organ of the abdomen is laboring under disease or injury it will soon affect the whole abdominal system.

Etiology and Treatment.—All irritations are effects of some cause. If so, is not a tumor an effect? What is the cause of its production? Why does it produce irritation? If the solar plexus is the center of the nervous system of the abdomen and if the great splanchnic nerve passing through the diaphragm to the solar plexus is the entire source of nutritive force to the abdominal viscera, have we not a paralysis of all the organs of the abdomen when we inhibit this supply of force and nourishment? Does paralysis of the organs of the abdomen follow such prohibition or inhibition? If this reasoning be true then we know why the abdominal artery forces blood into all organs of the abdomen in normal quantities and why the venous circulation whose nerves are affected fails to keep the organs in their normal condition by not carrying the waste venous blood and lymph from any organ as soon as this organ has received and appropriated its arterial blood.

We see at once that when the nerves of the veins become paralyzed the vein is inactive and full of venous blood that cannot pass on through the venous system normally. By this venous congestion we cause the arterial system to deposit the living arterial blood in the spongy membranes and it begins to construct flesh in an abnormal position and condition. Thus we reason that a tumor is the natural outgrowth of the living arterial blood when perverted from the normal functioning, and the appropriation of such blood which has been delivered to the organ but not carried away by venous return. I think this is why tumors are produced.

Two things in our system must be perfectly normal. First, the artery and its nerves must deliver constantly, on time and in quantity sufficient; second, the venous system and its nerves must perform their function and allow no accumulations. These two demands are absolute. The blood must go through and be delivered by the artery, and the venous system must carry the venous blood and all other substances back to the heart. Otherwise, tumors will appear as the result of such interference with the blood flow, either from or to the heart. On this foundation I see why we have tumors and why we have venous congestion. I think that to prohibit perfect freedom of the splanchnic nerve is to have partial paralysis of that division of the solar plexus which rules and governs both venous and arterial functioning to all organs of the abdomen.

Ask a mechanic what effect would follow the shutting off of the steam from a steam engine and his answer is "a universal stop or death." Ask him what would be the effect should you change the condition of the cam rod, or the head of the plunger. He would tell you that there would be palpitation of the heart. Throw a belt from any pulley and you will produce inaction at that point. Your saw wabbles because it is not properly adjusted on the mandrel. Without further details, I say you cannot expect to have good lumber cut with your engine and machine out of line. Take the square, plumb and level and line up all parts of the machinery that are necessary to cut good lumber. A tumor is a result. A belt is off and that organ suffers the loss of nerve and blood action. These remarks are intended for the mechanical brain of an osteopath with the advice that if he has none of the brains of a mechanic he had better quit because he will not comprehend the cause that has produced abnormal growths of any organ. He is at sea when consulted about these conditions unless he finds the shut-off or abnormality.

I never found a bed-wetting child or older person with both innominates and coccyx in proper position. I have never found enlargements or tumefactions of the uterus or ovaries with a perfectly normal articulation of the hip, sacrum, coccyx, lumbar and lower dorsal vertebrae. While the hip shows but little if any soreness at the joint, I have found in many of them luxations to a partial or complete dislocation from the socket. One says, what

159

has this to do with tumefaction of the organs of the pelvis and abdomen? Let me ask you if you should step on a nail and drive it through your foot why should you have lockjaw? Remember the jaw and foot are a great ways apart. We reason that a dislocated or strained hip, coccyx, sacrum, in nominate, lumbar vertebra or rib will produce an abnormal irritation, paralysis, stagnation, secondary growth of the uterus, kidneys, bladder or other organ. When consulted on such diseases it is wisdom to withhold your opinion until you have found the cause and know that you are right, then your advice will be good and to the point. To the mechanic all abnormalities are effects. This answers the whole question. Do not tell me you cannot put your fingers upon the cause.

In tumors of the uterus I have found abnormalities between the eighth dorsal and the coccyx, which have produced stagnation of nerve and blood force and local paralysis of the uterus and its appendages. I find a bad condition of a symphysis pubis, abnormal condition of the sacrum and one or both innominates. I often find the coccyx thrown from its normal position backwards, forwards or under, and producing disturbances of the sacral nerves pertaining to the uterus. I also find the ligaments and muscles surrounding the hip joints in a relaxed or constricted condition and producing much or little disturbance to the truly normal action of the whole excretory system of the pelvis, and back to the kidneys. I have no doubt from the good results obtained by correcting the coccyx, the innominates, the lumbar and the lower dorsal vertebrae, that we have demonstrated one of the greatest truths that the anatomical mechanic has ever gotten possession of, leading to a correct conclusion as to the cause and cure of an enlarged uterus and other lower abdominal tumors.

HERNIA.

Definition.—The protrusion of a loop or knuckle of an organ or tissue through an abnormal opening.

—*Dorland.*

Etiology and Treatment.—The meaning of the word hernia is so well understood that it is only necessary to say that such protrusions in the groin in the region of Poupart's ligament can easily be felt and seen. There is always some soreness in the region through which the bowels pass from the inner to the outer opening. The tumor grows larger, its soreness increases, the cord of the testicles becomes very tender and often enlarged as a result of the pressure and weight of the bowels above Poupart's ligament.

This irritation and tumor is the result of inhibition or temporary paralysis of the nerves that govern the blood supply of the ligaments, fascia and tissue in that region. Hydrocele is often found to precede the giving way of the fleshy substances in this region. These preceding symptoms appear in many cases before the tumor known as hernia begins to show up. I am speaking from practical experience of the irritation just above Poupart's ligament, for in my own case it existed at the beginning of the show of a small tumor upon myself which resulted in a hernia as large as an orange. I could reduce it with my hands; I wore all known kinds of trusses; I worked and worried with them for forty-two years before I took up the subject and reasoned as a mechanic should. Then I proceeded to make a truss with an oscillating wooden pad, by the use of which the orifice or opening of the hernia in my case and in other cases has healed or closed up.

I reasoned that an oval truss would enlarge the opening, and this I know is what follows the use of the ordinary truss which is oval. My truss consists of a small block of wood peculiar in shape and well understood only by seeing it. The wooden pad is about five inches in length and is so fastened to a single spring that it may turn in any direction that the body will take. The pad of wood, one spring, and a simple belt make up the truss, which will suit for either side. It holds the parts in place until the orifice heals up, in most cases of single hernia. My truss is perfectly comfortable to the person who wears it.

161

Surgeons have long since lost all confidence in the ability of any truss to do more than occasionally heal up the opening, and only after wearing them a long time. They resort to the use of the knife which in many cases I think avoidable. I think that many persons who have reducible hernias will be satisfied that my truss is a healer and not a source of annoyance.

Many cases operated on for appendicitis show no inflammation of the appendix when the opening is made with the knife and the appendix exposed. This soreness in the region of the appendix, which is mistaken for appendicitis, is often a premonitory symptom of a breach or hernia that will later make its appearance. My truss has proved this to be true because all soreness from either side disappears soon after the truss is applied. The osteopath should not be hasty in his diagnosis and say this is a case of appendicitis when it is simply the soreness in that region that accompanies the giving way of the parts previous to the appearance of a hernial tumor. The osteopath should acquaint himself with this fact else he will operate for appendicitis when there is but the coming of a hernia.

The osteopath should remember that sensible surgery is a part of osteopathy and his opinion if correct is good and if not correct will condemn his knowledge of cause and effect. A correct diagnosis will always vindicate our acquaintance with the structure of the human body, so let us be very careful and know that we are right in our opinion, particularly about appendicitis and hernias.

REGION ABOVE THE DIAPHRAGM

ABOVE THE DIAPHRAGM.

I have extended my study and exploration as a mechanic to the cause of diseases that prey upon the human system above the diaphragm. I have contended with all of the diseases of this division of the body. I have hunted for the cause or causes, and I know the question must be answered by the mechanic who is capable of exploring the blood and nerve supply from the heart to the brain.

I have found and demonstrated to my satisfaction, and think to the understanding of the qualified anatomist, that goiter is not a disease but an effect caused by an obstruction of both arterial and venous blood which produces a retention of the fluids that should be constantly returned to the heart through the venous system, without any obstruction. I find obstruction caused by both bone and muscle preventing the normal return of fluids and resulting in enlarged glands. I do not "suppose" this is the trouble because I see it as a self-evident fact. I have demonstrated this to myself when I have adjusted to the normal all parts that were abnormal or that would hinder a perfect flow of blood from and back to the heart, and have seen the goiter disappear. This demonstration vouches for the truth of this philosophy. I will now pass higher up with this method of reasoning, because I know that it applies, and will bear the skilled operator out and his reward is his success.

Diseases of the tonsils are an effect of pressure and constriction. Go on up to the submaxillary glands and all of those that you find enlarged and proceeding on to inflammation, and you will find that the obstructed blood which is prevented from entering the head to execute its normal work is busy building adenoids, polypi, nasal thickenings, and sometimes causing erysipelas, scarlet fever, diphtheria and so on. All of these abnormal growths and their effects follow obstruction to the normal flow of the fluids of the body. It matters not where the obstruction is, trouble follows.

If we do not know this law but use the knife, tongs, tweezers, and serums, we show that we do not know the producing cause. If we do not know this law, we should not proceed to operate. We may say that we can get more money by using our knife or tweezers for the removal of growths than we can get otherwise, but I will say that for many years I have made it my business to exhaust every other means of relief before I used the knife. My patient's recovery was more to me than the dollars. In my osteopathic work my object is to deliver arterial blood to its destination that it may execute all the physiological duties incumbent upon it. When it has finished the work of construction and re pair, then the next step or object that I have in view is to know that it returns to its shop to deliver its waste and be renewed. It did all it could while it was arterial blood, now it must be returned to the lungs to unite with new substances, receive atmosphere and go through all the qualifying processes necessary to the production of pure blood, and return to the heart that it may deliver arterial blood perpetually. Upon this life depends.

Now we will start from the heart towards the head with arterial blood for delivery at every station between the heart and the top of the head. I mean to deliver as much blood at each place as the normal requires and no more. Then the arterial blood must go on supplying station after station without obstruction until every organ including the brain is fully supplied and the blood has done its normal work of nourishing and rebuilding all the ordinary wear and tear, and must then return to the heart.

Now let me ask this question. Can this blood go from the heart to the top of the head when the muscles or tissues are contracted, especially in that locality through which the blood-vessels penetrate the skull? Should the heart fail to deliver the blood to the brain at this point—at the union of the neck with the head—could any man of reason see this stoppage and not know that congestion, irritation, stagnation and inflammation of the glandular system of this portion of the neck would result? He surely would know that in the glands, lymphatics and blood circulation there would be set up decomposition as a result of the blood retention. Then he has to deal with ear troubles, sore throat sore tonsils, sore larynx, sore pharynx, misery and chill, followed by fever.

Right here is the place where the medical doctor has stood confounded because he did not reason nor know the cause of the inflamed conditions which he calls by the name of croup, diphtheria, pharyngitis, laryngitis, grippe and so on. He dopes, doses and fails for the reason that he does not remove the cause as the mechanic would. Such has been the procedure for hundreds of years. It is the same today. To the physiological anatomist such diseases have no mystery, for as a mechanic he knows the cause; and in the treatment of such cases he should hold himself responsible for the results, at least when he has them in charge before a destruction of tissues or organs has taken place.

EPILEPSY.

Definition.—Falling sickness. Cerebrospinal disease, idiopathic or symptomatic, spontaneous or accidental, occurring in paroxysms; characterised by loss of consciousness and convulsive motions of the muscles, with uncertain intervals between the attacks. At times, before loss of consciousness occurs, a sensation as of a cold vapor is felt, hence called aura epileptica. It appears to rise in some part of the body, proceeds toward the head, and as soon as it has reached the brain the patient falls down. The ordinary duration of a fit is from five to twenty minutes, but it may be protracted for hours. In all cases there is loss of sensation, sudden falling down, distortion of the eyes and face; red, purple, or violet countenance; grinding of the teeth; foam ing at the mouth; convulsions of the limbs; difficult respiration, at times stertorous; with sometimes involuntary discharge of feces and urine. After the fit the patient may remain for some time affected with headache, stupor and lassitude. The disease is generally organic, but may be functional and symptomatic of irritation in other parts, as the stomach, bowels, etc. Prognosis as to ultimate recovery is unfavorable; the disease rarely destroys life, but may lead to mental imbecility. To attacks of epilepsy unaccompanied by convulsions the French gave the name of petit mal; they are preceded by vertigo, cerebral epilepsy. In the mildest cases the seizures are described as blanks, faints, forgets, absences, darknesses, etc., consciousness being, as it were, lost for a few seconds. Fully formed epilepsy is the grand mal of the French, spinal epilepsy. When furious mania succeeds a paroxysm it is termed mania epileptica and epileptic delirium.

—Dunglison.

Etiology.—We have given you Dunglison's definition which about covers the whole ground of the condition known as epilepsy. You see by this definition that in medication there is but little hope for eradication and recovery from this so-called disease. To the medical doctor this disease is now and always has been an unsolved mystery in so far as its cause is concerned. Having known this for many years I concluded that here medication was a failure. I worked with medicine and treated my patients with such remedies as are used in such cases, but without avail. Then I began to reason and hunt for anatomical malpositions of the human framework which could in any manner obstruct the natural functioning of either blood or nerve system.

We generally find in the history of such patients that they have at some time suffered some injury. For instance, they have been thrown from a horse, have fallen from a tree, from a house, down stair-ways, into the cellar, or in some manner they have had a heavy fall, head and shoulders striking the ground first, and on examination I have universally found either a dislocated atlas, axis, some joint of the neck or some rib or dorsal vertebra, and sometimes as low down as the lumbar. Some of them are thrown out of their normal position and interfere with blood and nerve circulation. I believe all such spasms are the result of an impoverished spinal cord from the medulla to the diaphragm.

Treatment.—In treating patients suffering with epilepsy, I generally place a stool twelve or fourteen inches high on the floor and have my patient kneel before it and lay his chest upon it in order to have his spine on a level with the stool. Then, as I have so often told you, I stand behind him and with my knees grasp his hips firmly while I thoroughly manipulate his spine from the fifth lumbar up. I then proceed to adjust all variations in every joint from the occiput to the lumbar, both spine and ribs. I want the entire spinal nervous system as well as the whole of the sympathetic to be absolutely free from obstruction of any kind whatsoever that could in any manner arise from any misplaced bone or contracted muscle. The blood and nerve supply to the entire nervous system must be free and unobstructed. Once or twice a week is often enough to treat these epileptic patients. As to diet, the ordinary plain food is good enough, but never permit your patient to go to bed with a heavily loaded stomach. Such patients should stir around for at least two to four hours before bed time. Remember this, keep all drugs out of these patients. In many cases I have had more difficulty to get my patient out from under the poisonous effects of drugs than I had to remove the cause of the disease. For the encouragement of the osteopath I will say that there is hope not only for relief but for cure in many cases. I have given permanent relief to many patients and some relief to all.

INSANITY AND FEEBLENESS OF MIND, OR MENTAL SHORTAGE OR OVERPLUS.

Definition. Insanity.—Disorder of the mental faculties, more or less permanent in character, but without loss of consciousness and will. It is marked by delusions, illusions, and hallucinations, by changes in character and habits, and by unreasonable and purposeless actions and language.

—*Dorland.*

Definition. Idiocy.—Complete congenital imbecility; extreme dementia.

—*Dorland.*

Definition. Idiot—A fool; a person without understanding.

—*Dorland.*

We have two known conditions before us. First, an abnormal shortage in mental forces and supply which results in feebleness of mind, or idiocy. Second, we have extreme mental vehemence of all grades which results in insanity and suicide with all their horrors.

The leaders in the healing art have philosophized and experimented with drugs, physical punishment, using the whip and other instruments of cruelty upon the unfortunate with abnormal minds, without restoring them to normal mentality. After experimenting with poisonous and harmless drugs, the doctor proceeds to the post-mortem, hoping that he may find cause for this effect. He analyzes the blood and other fluids; he opens the head and takes out the brain and with his microscope he scrutinizes all divisions of it and reports that to all appearances the brain is absolutely normal and that he has found no known cause for the abnormality of brain action. About the same opinion has been given not alone by medical doctors but by the doctors of all schools. They report their conclusion to be that the causes producing such abnormal conditions are absolutely unknown; and they chain the maniac to a post or place him in a cell in order to protect themselves and others from injury. I do not claim to be the philosopher who has solved the question of insanity, its cause and its remedy, but I do claim that for many years I have made myself familiar with others' opinions about the treatment of maniacs and idiots. From all I have seen and read I am fully satisfied that the world is a total blank on this subject and would be just as well off without a line that has been written on it.

Etiology.—Knowing the above to be true I will ask, will we still dope, dose, torture and confine the insane and say, verily, verily, the grave is the only asylum that will cure such diseases? Is the mechanical philosopher satisfied to cast his vote and give his consent with the world that there is no hope to bring the man back from insanity to normal mental action by hunting for a physical cause that has produced bony variations from their normal articulation which results in shortage or overplus in the supply of some one or more of the five senses—seeing, hearing, feeling, smelling, and tasting?

Isn't there a shortage or overplus of cerebrospinal fluid or some other substance that should be normally delivered to what is known as the sympathetic ganglia or system? Are these fluids delivered to their destination on time and in quantity to suit the demand of the whole nervous system? Are not the five senses inseparably connected with the emotions and are they not subordinate to mentality? Is not the business of the cardiac center to control any overpluses from the nutrient ganglion and keep down emotional excesses?

In the human body there are five systems of nerves that must be normal and in the very best of health so as to do their full duty. They are the motor, nutrient, sensory, emotional and mental. There are five kinds of nerves in the sensory system. They are the nerves of sight, smell, taste, hearing, feeling, and all should obey the demand of the mental system. The sensory system gives notice to the mental what it sees, hears, smells, tastes and feels, and then the mind, or mental system gives orders just what to do. If there is danger near, the motor system is ordered to move and preserve the body. If the motor fails to obey the order to move or run, then death or injury to the body may follow. Thus life depends on obedience of the motor nerve division.

All mental orders are based upon the favorable or um favorable report of one or more of the five sensory sets of nerves. So we see at once that mentality or the mind of man, in all its action has as its foundation for its conclusions the report or reports of one or more of the five senses. If the mind is normal then wise conclusions and judicious orders are issued for the support and comfort of the human body. But suppose we have a break—a diseased, wounded or disabled condition of the motor nerve—then we will have a failure in perfect obedience to the orders of the mental system. Suppose the nutrient system should fail to nourish any division or the whole body, the result is prostration either of the division or of the whole body. Any confusion or failure in the whole nerve system or in any division will show imperfection in health, mental or physical action, just in proportion to the shortage, or injuries received.

Would the mechanic say he thinks the friction known as insanity can be traced to the nerves of the five senses? The five senses make their report to the superior ruler of the emotions which is mentality. I am satisfied that in many cases a mechanical critic in search for the cause of diseased mentality will find wounds of the head such as are made by clubs, beer bottles and shocks of other kinds that would produce abnormality of brain action. In other cases he will find strains and dislocations of the neck and the dorsal somewhere between the atlas and the diaphragm of such a degree as to disable the healthy action of mentality. Then, because of the disabled condition of mentality the emotional becomes the ruler. Thus we have a cause for rash acts. Whenever mentality is not powerful enough to control the emotional we have the condition known as insanity. So the army of life fails to accomplish its work because of a diseased commander—Mentality.

In dissecting the bodies of maniacs, I have found abnormal positions and conditions of the bones from the atlas to the tenth dorsal, and ossified joints of the cervical region, also some of the upper dorsal. As a mechanic wishing to relieve diseased mentality, I confine my labors and reasoning to mechanical causes and physiological effects. I have found two or three bones united by ossifications. I have found the results of all grades of inflammatory conditions of the spinal cord. I have found ribs twisted off their articulations with the transverse processes, twisted and turned under and into the spaces above and below their articulation. I have found enlarged spinal columns, nearly every joint from diaphragm to coccyx enlarged. Such conditions are usually accompanied by renal calculi and all grades of kidney disease. I am satisfied that these abnormalities have much to do with insanity, tuberculosis, shaking palsy, hysteria, epilepsy, locomotor ataxia and many other diseases. I think these variations produce fermentation of the venous blood and continue this yeast forming process on which the body must then depend for its nourishment. Since the birth of Osteopathy in 1874, I have sought and hunted faithfully to find the cause, or friction, that produces such abnormal conditions as are seen in the raving maniac. I am satisfied if the cause is ever found, it will be found by the genius of the mechanical philosopher, and the answer will be—friction. Is this friction or disturbance in the nerve centers and branches of the neck and upper dorsal region? Mechanical variations of this region produce confused action and abnormal work of the nutrient ganglion and the motor and nutrient centers of the cardiac plexus. I think the mechanic who is qualified to find the cause of friction that produces insanity will be the Columbus who has discovered the new world or continent of which sanity, peace and harmony of mind and body are the inhabitants.

Treatment.—It is the work of the mechanic to adjust all bony variations, all mechanical or obstructing causes of any kind that would prohibit the easy transit of blood to and from the heart, also nerve fluid and force to and from the brain. It is his business to keep up perpetual harmony both in blood and nerve supply.

SHAKING PALSY.

Definition. Paralysis Agitans.—Shaking palsy, trembling palsy; variety of tremor in which the muscles are in a perpetual alternation of contraction and relaxation, often accompanied by incoordination.

—*Dunglison.*

Shaking palsy is a mountain that the doctors of all schools have failed to climb. I have been very careful to peruse many authors on this subject. I have spent years in hearing doctors discuss it, and I am frank to say that so far I have not found or heard a word, sentence or chapter which gave me any light on the cause producing shaking palsy.

I laid down the books of theories, practice, diagnosis, prognosis, and treatment because I could see nothing that would be of any benefit to the afflicted man or woman. Then I began to reason that there was a mechanical cause for this effect, and came to the conclusion that the mechanic was governed by law in his reasoning from effect to cause, and from him I would get some truth on the subject.

Etiology.—I reason that a well-fed horse always shows normal action of the whole system, and that if the horse is not fed, watered, well stabled, or if it is strained by overloading, I could expect to see in it such an effect or condition of tremulous motions, as is found in shaking palsy. I reasoned that a horse would generally come out of this tremulous condition if his system be well nourished, watered, and given a reasonable amount of rest. A muscle, nerve or blood-vessel should be nourished and cared for with the same wisdom that a veterinarian would use in the handling of a horse placed in his care.

On examination, with a view of finding, if possible, the cause producing shaking palsy, I have found vertebrae in the lower half of the neck or the upper dorsal partially dislocated, and also that the first, second, third and fourth ribs, one or more, were out of place. The facets of one or more of these vertebrae were in an abnormal position and locked against the other facet of the articulation. The shoulder blade, the collar bone, the ribs and vertebrae as low down as the eighth dorsal, that is, the shoulder and all the bones thereunto belonging, are brought down and held together by spasmodic contracture of the muscles of the axillary region. As a mechanic I thought I could see here a cause that produces dwarfage of the whole system from the eighth dorsal to the atlas. On all cases that I have examined, I have found absolute and indisputable derangement of the spine, ribs, scapulae and clavicles, finding them drawn from their normal articulation by this continued contraction of muscles. There is plenty of evidence to show the osteopathic mechanic that shaking palsy is an effect of a cause producing atrophy of the whole system from the eighth rib to the atlas, by shutting off the blood, cerebrospinal and other fluids that should nourish the nervous system.

Prognosis.—Until I can remove the cause of the suspension of nerve and other vital fluids and restore a normal blood supply I have no hope of giving temporary nor permanent relief. This is all that I can say as to the prognosis of this serious condition which has stood before the philosophers of the world for thousands of years without their having asked, where is the cut off? With what I have said and your knowledge of anatomy and physiology, we can hope for success if we remove all obstructions to nerve and blood supply.

When I have a case of paralysis agitans of long standing and affecting the arms I know it is a very serious condition giving but little hope of complete recovery. Abnormal conditions existing in the spine and ribs have obstructed the normal supply to the intercostal arteries and nerves, and by long starvation have caused the nervous system above the diaphragm to become feeble and almost obliterated. I only hope to give relief and some strength to the nerves of nutrition. We can expect to palliate the symptoms in proportion to nutrition being re-established by a proper adjustment.

Examination.—In your examination find where the nerves are impinged, or the blood supply to the cord and muscles and the drainage from them are hindered. To satisfy yourself on this subject begin your search for the cause first at the atlas, then continue on down through all of the joints of the neck and the dorsal as low as the ninth. Search carefully to know that each vertebra is in place and in true articulation with its accompanying ribs, so that no-muscle will be irritated sufficiently to produce a contracture. In all the cases of paralysis agitans which have come to me for examination and treatment I have found a badly deformed spine, being either anterior, convex or in abnormal lateral position.

Examine carefully the muscles of the neck, especially the scaleni, which are usually found atrophied, shortened, and irritated to such a degree as to result in the nodding motion of the head. Then go to the lower cervical vertebrae to make sure there is no impingement on the lower cervical nerves or blood-vessels in that region such as would result in irritation, contraction and a trembling effort of the muscles to remove the impingement. Examine carefully the intercostal spaces of the eight upper ribs of both sides to see that those ribs are not turned or out of normal articulation.

I will give an account of my own case. When on a Santa Fe train going at the rate of a mile a minute we ran into a freight that was standing on the main track. I was lying in the berth with my head towards the engine. My head struck hard against the head-board of the berth and hurt my spine from the atlas to the eighth dorsal, and left all the ribs on my left side on a heavy strain, and the fifth and sixth were thrown out and above the articulation on the transverse processes.

In two or three months afterwards I had shaking palsy of my head and neck. I examined the union of the seventh cervical with the first dorsal and found the facets on the upper surface of the first dorsal were shoved to the right on the under facets of the lower cervical which were slipped sideways and almost off from the facets of the upper dorsal. The under surfaces of the second dorsal facets were almost pushed off the upper surfaces of the third. I took my walking cane which is bent so as to form a hook for a hand-hold. I fastened this cane in a vice and brought the hook-end down below the bulge that was o-n my neck and with great force I pulled back until the lock was separated. After adjusting my neck I proceeded to have my ribs as low down as the eighth on the left side adjusted, and the shaking of my head stopped. On examining others I find about the same condition of neck, spine and ribs. Upon careful examination of the vertebrae of the cervical and upper dorsal the student will see at once that all the facets have a limit of motion, a stopping place. When thrown by force strong enough to disarticulate the facets to the right, left or backwards from the absolutely normal, we have a condition that the muscles labor to overcome, a condition that will produce shaking palsy.

Treatment.—When called upon to treat a case of paralysis agitans you must understand that you have a machine that is out of order at some point where it interferes with the nerve and blood supply to the posterior scaleni muscles. You must find the exact region of the shut-off and adjust the misplacement, and let the blood and nerve supply have unobstructed action in delivering their fluids to repair wasted or starved tissues and the nerves of motion and nutrition.

Where does this blood or nerve force come from? What arteries are involved? Seek the branch given off from the large vessels that supply the neck muscles and make sure there is nothing to hinder the normal flow of blood. To give freedom to the intercostal blood and nerve supply work to correct all of the dorsal vertebrae as low down as the ninth, both in their articulation with each other and with the ribs on both sides. Adjust carefully the inferior maxilla drawing it well forward and off the superior cervical ganglion and the blood-vessels that lie just back of its angle.

The more thoroughly we study and understand our anatomy and physiology the better we are prepared to proceed as engineers in these cases and the more successful will be our work. As the osteopath is well posted in adjusting the upper dorsal vertebrae I will be brief here and say that I prefer to have my patient seated while I stand before him, then I pass my right arm under the patient's left arm and extend it across his back and bring my fingers in a hooked manner over the upper ribs of his right side and bring them down to place. In treating the opposite or left side I pass my left arm across the patient's breast and under the patient's right arm and reverse the treatment. Do this on both sides so as to loosen up the muscles that are obstructing the flow of blood.

In my observation I have no memory of ever seeing a man with shaking palsy who used crutches. After normalizing the spine and ribs I say to my afflicted patient, get you a pair of crutches and use them. Throw as much weight of the body on the crutches as possible. Use them with moderation indoors and out of doors every day. With your weight on the crutches spend as much time as possible in the open air. Also use them in the house because when in the house the flesh or muscles relax, and to hang the weight of the body on the crutches will give a great advantage to the intercostal nerves and blood-vessels. The weight of the body on the crutches will assist in keeping the ribs in place.

Follow this method of treatment for a few months and if you realize that the nutrient system is gaining by such treatment keep on and on as long as you get good results. Be very careful to always keep a good flow of blood between the ribs through the intercostal arteries and veins as well as through the entire axillary system. Stand your patient in the doorway with his back against the jamb of the door, then put your hands on the patient's shoulders and gently press them out ward and upward in order to free up the scapulae. This will give the nerves and blood in the scapular and axillary regions some chance for normal circulation. The operator should give his attention once or twice a week to the neck, back, shoulders and arm pits. Continue your treatment throughout the lumbar region in order to give as much relief as is possible to the lower limbs which are usually affected.

TORTICOLLIS.

Definition.—Stiffneck, wryneck. A form of muscular rheumatism, seated in the neck, which prevents the motion of the head and causes the patient to hold it inclined to the side affected. It is commonly of short duration, usually disappearing in a few days. Also permanent contraction of the muscles of the neck, torticollis spastica, which causes the head to be held to one side.

—Dunglison.

Etiology.—After having carefully examined such cases as have come to me during the last thirty years, it is my opinion that torticollis has such etiologic factors as imperfect articulation of one or more of the cervical facets on one side of the neck. I found that the lower end of one of the outer facets had been pulled up so high as to let it fall inside of the upper edge of the inner facet with which it should articulate. This condition causes irritation and a thickening and shortening of the muscles which produces a gradual but continued contraction. Thus is produced and maintained a permanent dislocation.

Many causes tend to produce luxations or dislocations of the neck, chief among which is an unskillful use of forceps at the time of extracting teeth; such mechanical injuries to the cervical region as occur in collisions on railroads where the head is brought with great force against a wall or a berth; also other abrupt stops of the body such as would tend to throw the head suddenly and violently backward from the body; falls down stairs or from horseback (especially of children and aged people); carrying heavy weights on head or shoulders; the manner some children have of jumping suddenly forward and into the back of a playmate resulting in a quick backward jerk of the head. There is often a permanent dislocation the effects of which are the many abnormal conditions of the neck that we see and which often manifest far-reaching results.

Prognosis.—The prognosis of wryneck is very favorable when it is taken in hand in its early stage. The chronic form can be very greatly benefited. The mechanical skill of the osteopath here aids him to readjust dislocations of the neck just as well as any other portion of the body. When bony adhesions have not taken place the osteopath can adjust the bones and do much good and give relief to the contractured muscles. Correct articulation followed by normal action has been the result of my observation and work in many cases. When you find bony adhesions I would advise you to let such cases alone for they are surgical.

Examination.—We must remember that in such conditions as wryneck, or torticollis, we have a call for our mechanical skill. I consider these effects are such as follow luxations or dislocations, partial or complete, and in order that the exploration or searching for the cause producing any one of the effects above described be made thorough, place your patient upon the table on his back. Then most carefully examine every structure on both sides of the neck from the seventh cervical on up to and including the articulation of the atlas with the base of the skull in order to ascertain whether or not the facets of the vertebrae are in true position. In some cases I have found the atlas too far back at one end or process and too far forward at the other.

See that each cervical vertebra is in its normal position and not turned and holding the muscles of the upper portion of the neck in a twisted condition producing irritation and such contractures as often follow. Examine carefully the ligamentum nuchae in all its parts. Go to the lower articulations of the first and second dorsal vertebrae and know for a certainty that no rib has been driven by fall, strain or otherwise from its normal position so as to interfere by misplacement or pressure with the blood or nerve supply to the neck.

Treatment.—Place your patient on his back on the table with his head near the upper end. Then standing at his head begin your work upon the cervical vertebrae. Carefully test and make sure of every articulation. Draw your patient about six inches beyond the end of the table, bring pressure to bear upon the head down toward the body in order that the muscles of the neck can become loosened or shortened. Place the fingers of one hand on the under side of the neck to steady the transverse processes then place the other fingers on the processes just above and with a gentle rotatory motion move the neck so as to give freedom to the muscles which are held tight or irritated.

Remember that the neck is not always dislocated when held tight by irritation, but the muscles have been thrown so far back that they cannot return to their normal position without assistance. Thus you will see that your work is to readjust the muscles and permit the articulations to return to normal. Remember that the ligamentum nuchae is often put on such a strain by luxation as to produce a drawing of the head to one side. It is necessary that while we have the head pressed back so as to bend the neck and loosen the posterior muscles of the neck and nuchae that we draw the nuchae up into place. You will often be surprised to have the whole cervical system fall into line and give quick relief. While in this position it is sometimes necessary to move the neck back and forth from right to left in order to loosen it up.

I want to caution the operator that when we pull or twist the neck of these patients we must use but little force, just enough to loosen the muscles, because in many such cases the muscles on one or the other side of the neck are tight and on a strain and are likely to be held there by bony locks or adhesions. Should you find the seventh cervical vertebra too far back or forward on the first dorsal (a lesion which operates as a cause of the rheumatic soreness of the muscles), adjust that and you get relief. When your case is of a chronic nature, require your patient to come to you but once each week. You will soon find the results of your work will be the better because Nature has meanwhile been given a chance to repair the disordered condition.

I think I have said enough here for the operator to comprehend that he must use the best skill of a mechanic in his work of treating stiff necks if he hopes for good results. Be careful and stop when your patient says "you hurt my neck." Change your fingers, as you may be holding down a muscle which would come slack by taking your fingers off. In my experience the results of such treatment have been good. I have never advised the use of the knife, never having found it necessary. I think it far better to give what relief you can than to mutilate your patient.

OBESITY.

Definition.—Polysarcia. Excessive corpulence.

—Dunglison.

What is obesity? What causes this over-accumulation of fat? What nerves are at fault? Is it the sensory, motor or nutrient ganglion that has failed to do its duty? Have the arterial system and its nerves failed to do their duty, or have we paralysis of the nutrient system which belongs to the arterial nerves? As an engineer please answer these questions. An intelligent answer is expected of us.

What is the difference between obesity and diabetes? Is diabetes the result of venous and lymphatic action producing an abnormal flow of fluids from the body? If so, where is the break that produces irritation of the excretory nerves of the whole system? Does it produce an irritation of the sympathetic ganglia which perverts normal functioning and causes the system and kidneys to receive and pass off so much water? Do the lungs assist the excretories? Do they produce water and supply the excretory system? What is wrong in the machinery producing this condition? Diabetes and obesity are effects following heavy subluxations in the region of first, second, third and fourth upper dorsal. In that region we have sensation, motion and nutrition to consider. These questions are intended to make you hunt for a cause and then give us an answer by which we can proceed to deliver the patient from either diabetes or obesity. Diabetes is a continuous waste of the substances of the body that should be appropriated to normal form and motion. In obesity we have just the reverse condition. The arteries deliver the nutrient substances but the nerves of nutrition fail to receive and appropriate for normal purposes. Thus we have a piling up of a great quantity of unappropriated fat and other chemical substances in the system that should have been used by the nutrient system.

Etiology.—I think the deposit of fatty substances is the result of the fuel being brought to the furnace for living force and heat and not being consumed. Fat should be used as is necessary to run the engine of life and to build the normal, and the overplus should be thrown off. What would an engineer think or do in case his furnace would not consume and appropriate

181

fuel for the heat and action of his boiler, engine and machinery? When a man or woman comes to me for counsel and advice for the reduction of this rubbish or overplus I reason that there was an object for the production of this oil; it is as much a fuel for the furnace of life as coal is for the steam engine. Why has it not been consumed and appropriated normally?

I conclude there is an abnormal variation of some of the vertebrae or ribs that have interfered with the consumption of this fat or fuel and with the production of the force that should have been produced by it. As a result the engine is weak and helpless in its constructive power and its power to carry off the debris. The abdomen, heart and lungs being undisturbed bring the food for use, and because it is not used the tissues store up an overplus. When deposited it is a live substance, and not being consumed it remains as a weighty overplus.

In all fat persons I have examined in thirty years I find the spinous processes of the first and second dorsal vertebrae posterior to the processes of the third and fourth and tilted upward. I also find the lower vertebrae of the neck pulled forward. The lower ends of the scapulae are spread away from the spine while the upper ends are pulled towards the spine. The clavicles are far back and often on top of their articulating processes. This condition of the bones produces pressure on the inferior cervical, the sympathetic ganglia, and the pneumogastric nerves. With this condition we cannot expect healthy action of the lungs, heart, arteries, veins and nerves which should prepare, appropriate and consume nutriment, renovate the body and keep it in normal form and functioning condition.

Treatment.—My object is to adjust the parts of the framework to their normal relations, making it impossible for undue pressure to interfere with the power of the nerves to drive the blood through all parts, to deliver and construct, or to interfere with the blood in picking up and carrying away all waste substances in such a manner that normal functioning is the result.

I commence my treatment in the neck or upper dorsal. The first and second dorsal are pushed far back on the body of the third with the spinous processes sticking up and backwards very prominently, which brings heavy pressure upon the motor nerves; thus we have paralysis of the nutrient nerves of the upper dorsal. The failure of the second dorsal to articulate properly with the third is the point I seek to normalize in order that nutrition be consumed.

Then you will have force and action instead of inactivity and excessive weight. Sometimes I place my patient upon his back, bring his scapulae to the head end of the treating table and with the patient's head resting on my arms I place the fingers of both hands on the transverse processes of the involved vertebra; then I move the head and neck from side to side bending the spine enough to unlock the articulations. Exert pressure to keep the muscles relaxed while you correct the lesion. I will give you another good method. While the person is sitting in a chair bring the sternum forward and against your knee, your foot being on the chair and between the man's legs. If a lady, the foot may be placed beside her. The object is to make a fixed point for the breast to lean against. Then bend the head and neck down over your knee, giving lateral movements on neck and upper dorsal to the right and left. Hold the fingers firmly over the dorsal processes. Then with the hand under the chin raise the head up and back with a view of getting normal articulation of the facets of the upper vertebrae.

With patient face downward on the table adjust the lumbar region and the dorsal up to the fourth. While patient is still in this position, with the heels of the hands work solidly downward on the ribs and spines that are too much covered with flesh and fat. Before leaving your patient be careful to adjust the clavicles and scapulae. My object is normality at every point of articulation of spine and ribs, from the atlas to the sacrum. Generally I treat such cases twice a week. I have had good success in the reduction of fat in such cases, and I hope others will follow it up. My object has been to make the machinery consume and appropriate that which is necessary, and throw off the remainder. I want the lungs, skin and kidneys each to do its part in the work of excretion. If the machine is in a truly normal condition you may expect to find solidity of flesh instead of the fat, flabby condition.

HODGKIN'S DISEASE.

Definition.—Glandular sarcoma, lymph adenoma pseudoleukemia. A chronic disease mainly characterized by the enormous enlargement of the lymphatic glands of the body, along with a peculiar deposit in the spleen, and accompanied by a pernicious anemia. * * * The prognosis is unfavorable.

—Dunglison.

Etiology.—About all the information concerning Hodgkin's disease that we get from medical and surgical literature is simply the effects, the progress and the termination, which, as all of the authors agree, is death within a few years. I have bulked the medical and surgical conclusions with Dunglison's definition of this disease and find that by medication there is no hope. All describe the extensive glandular enlargement but give no clue to the cause or causes producing it. Surgical interference offers no hope or expectation of cure.

In 1874 I began to reason that suspended nerve action and obstructed blood and lymphatic circulation were the causes of enlarged thyroid, deep and superficial cervical, axillary and mammary lymphatic glands. Because of the results following my work in this line I have been very much encouraged to continue my investigation. I have worked out my belief that the nerve and blood circulations are obstructed before the appearance of such glandular conditions.

I discovered that the reduction of the enlarged glands to their normal size was the result that followed a properly adjusted bony system, especially the spine from the occiput to the ninth dorsal vertebra, and the ribs, clavicles, scapulae, hyoid and inferior maxillary bones. I put them each and every one in a condition that would take off all restraint from a perfect circulation. I was not only surprised but was placed as I considered it upon a firm foundation to reason back to the cause that produced such effects, for with every few exceptions, success followed my treatment which was confined to the one object—to obtain perfect freedom for both nerve and blood supply from the brain and heart to all the parts affected, and an unobstructed venous return.

When I have a case of glandular enlargement I ask my patients to roll up their sleeves, and as I expect, they show me vaccine scars which are generally large and deep and the report is that there was much suffering during their development. From my observations I reason that the vaccine virus or poison which is still retained in the system is in these cases showing its effects in connection with the glandular enlargement and has done its part in weakening the powers of renovation in the whole glandular system. If you will allow me to digress a little I will say that in my observation there has been a wonderful increase of tuberculosis since vaccination has had a legal inforcement.

Treatment.—I have never found a glandular enlargement above the diaphragm unless I found much abnormality in location and position of the facets and articulations of the vertebrae, the ribs and the bones of the neck. I believe this abnormality is the cause that produces such effects as are seen in Hodgkin's disease and in my treatment I govern myself according to this philosophy.

As a mechanic I begin my explorations at the atlas. In almost every case of enlarged glands of the neck both deep and superficial I have found the atlas in an abnormal position. This I adjust being very careful to know that its articulation with the occiput is absolutely correct. I then adjust the other bones of the neck. I often find the seventh cervical abnormal in its articulation with the first dorsal. This I carefully correct and proceed with my examination very thoroughly as far down as the tenth dorsal adjusting every abnormality found. Often I find a lateral curvature of a very serious nature which should be corrected. Then I go to the clavicles and examine them at each end because in many of these glandular enlargements I have found the clavicles too far back and under or above the acromian processes. When such is the case I proceed to bring them forward into place on the acromian process and also adjust their articulations with the sternum.

I am very particular to know that the manubrium is correct in its articulation with the gladiolus and that all ribs above the diaphragm are in their proper places articulating as they should. After this is done I raise the arm up in a perpendicular position and adjust the scapulae which are very often found in the abnormal condition known as "winged scapulae." I return them to their natural position by adjusting the outer end of the clavicle in its articulation with the acromian process.

Without squeezing or in any way irritating these glands I place my hands below them and gently but firmly draw them up in order to give better

185

circulation to their nerve and blood supply. The flat of the hand can be gently brought to bear for a while on these glands when they have been so lifted up but no rough gouging with the points of your fingers is necessary while you are giving this glandular treatment.

DISEASES OF THE SWEAT GLANDS.

Definitions. Hidrosis.—Cutaneous disease accompanied with disturbance of the function of the sudoriferous apparatus.

Anhidrosis.—Deficient or absent secretion of sweat.

Hyperhidrosis.—Excessive sweating.

Bromidrosis.—Fetid sweat.

Sudamina.—Small vesicles appearing upon the skin, especially in the summer time, in hot countries, and in diseases attended with much sweating; sweat vesicles. It is a military eruption.

—Dunglison.

Etiology.—I have always looked for the cause of such effects as are seen in either deficient or profuse sweating of the hands, the feet, the axilla of any one part, or of the entire body and I consider them to be the result of temporary or continued paralysis of the nerves which control the sweat glands of the entire body, or some portion of it. In many cases I think this condition follows vaccination, whooping-cough, measles, tonsillitis pneumonia and all such diseases as temporarily or permanently derange the nerve and blood supply of the lymphatics of the superficial fascia.

We should be particular to restore the parts to their normal nerve action which means for the skin to both secrete and excrete. I think it is just as important for the glands to secrete from the atmosphere as it is for them to excrete to the atmosphere. To excite excretion and to suspend secretion is to have an abnormality, an overplus of sweat.

Examination.—We should make it our business in all such cases to very carefully explore the entire spine beginning with the atlas. I have found some necks very abnormal, some were lateral, some anterior, others posterior. Either the atlas, the axis or some other vertebra in the neck is likely to be out of its natural articulation. In some cases the inferior maxillary bone is at fault. From this point we go on with our explorations from the bones of the neck to those of the dorsal portion of the spine. We hunt for variations from the first to the twelfth dorsal then on through the lumbar to the sacrum and coccyx in order to ascertain where the nerve supply is interfered with.

Authorities vary in their opinions about the exact location of the sweat centers, some thinking the most important center is located in the medulla, while others think the centers are located in various parts of the nervous system. I will not dispute with the writers about what they have acknowledged they do not understand, but I will agree with them and go further, and take all of the brain and the entire nervous system, and then I know I am in possession of all nerve centers and branches and I proceed with my treatment. In short, we must neither have excitement by irritation nor prostration by inhibition of the nerves of the skin or superficial fascia if we expect healthy action of the system of sweat glands.

Treatment.—When a patient comes to me suffering from a perverted condition of the sweat glandular system, without hesitation I proceed to examine the whole spinal system of bones beginning with the coccyx. We should be very careful to know that this work is thoroughly done and that every part is left in normal condition, because an irritation at some point will produce contraction of the secretory system and at the same time put in action the excretory glands. After leaving the coccyx I am just as careful to seek and obtain perfect adjustment of the innominates and the sacrum. After this I take up the lumbar and adjust every section of that region. Then I most carefully explore and adjust every vertebra from there on up the spine to the atlas. I am careful to have perfect articulation of the ribs with the transverse processes of the spine. Now I continue my work in the region of the axilla and am particularly careful to have the articulations of the clavicle with the sternum and scapulae perfect.

I generally have my patient take the knee-chest position, chest on stool about twelve inches high, and proceed with my spinal treatment thoroughly from the sacrum to the dorsal. Give this treatment as I have described it in other chapters. Then I have my patient lie at full length on the treating table, face down, and with the heel of my hand I rub quite hard the entire length of the spine. I do this in order that I may loosen up the fascia all over the back. I work with a quick strong motion so as to have the back very hot from the friction of my hand as it passes over it.

This treatment I give twice each week with good results. I think any good operator by following out what I have indicated will get the result of normal glandular action in the part affected whether it be the axilla, the hands or the feet. My success has been very satisfactory. In cases of unilateral sweating of the face, when examining for cause I have usually found the atlas too far forward towards the angle of the inferior maxilla. Also there was a subluxation of the inferior maxilla which was displaced backwards and pressing on the facial nerve and interfering with the normal action of the superior cervical ganglion. To relieve this condition I place the fingers of one hand on the front side of the transverse processes of the atlas and upper cervical vertebrae and the fingers of the other hand behind the angle of the jaw and gently pull the atlas back and the jaw forward. This frees the blood and nerve circulation. I think this will enable the operator to successfully treat such patients as come to him suffering with disordered sweat glands.

STAMMERING OR STUTTERING.

Definition of Stammer.—To utter words with hesitation or imperfectly. To articulate imperfectly, to mispronounce certain letters as in rhotacism, lisping, etc.

—Dunglison.

Definition of Stuttering.—Interrupted and impeded articulation, due to spasms of the muscles of respiration, phonation, and articulation—one or all. As usually employed it is practically synonymous with stammering, but writers have endeavored to establish a distinction between the two words, employing stuttering to denote a hesitating speech dependent upon difficulty in enunciating syllables beginning with a consonant, and stammering to denote the habitual mispronunciation of certain letters. Rhotacism and lisping are forms of stammering in this sense.

—Dunglison.

Etiology.—When the first case of stammering came to me for osteopathic treatment, my observation was such as to lead me to the conclusion that the vocal and the respiratory nerves were brought too close together, thus the confusion in the expression of words. In all stammering cases which I have observed and treated during the many years past I have found without exception that my patient tried to talk with empty lungs. This gives a chance for the vocal and respiratory nerves to come too close together. A telegrapher would say "the wires are crossed." With this philosophy in mind I sought the demonstration of its truthfulness. While I have not had a very great number of stammering patients I have succeeded in giving those I have had perfect freedom from this embarrassing condition.

Treatment.—I have never found any specific bony lesions in stammering patients, yet minor ones can exist. I generally began at the atlas and explored and adjusted not only the cervical vertebrae but also the hyoid bone, the clavicles and the upper ribs bringing them all into as near a normal condition as was possible. After this was gently but thoroughly done the patient's work began. I would say to him "take a good big breath. Fill your lungs just as full as they can possibly hold then repeat each word after me clearly and distinctly

190

as I call them over. Now fill and say-one; fill and say two; fill and say three." Let them count on up to ten or fifteen. Then I would say, "load up your lungs, get them very full and say, man; load up and say, woman."

For the first day I would have them load up the lungs before every word spoken, my object being to separate the vocal and respiratory nerves by having the lungs very full of atmospheric air and just ready to blow out, so that each nerve could perform its function normally. When I drilled my patient two, three or more times a day I would have him distinctly with full lungs, pronounce two words such as "North America." The next lesson three words. By this time I have him so that he can fill the lungs and speak sentences of four or five words such as "I want you to stop." "I want you to trot," or some such phrases.

For some time I kept my patient close to me not allowing him to speak to any other person but myself and I cautioned him not to try to answer any person or pronounce any word until his lungs were so full they were ready to blow off. By this process at the end of a week or ten days I would discharge my patient with the order positively never to speak until he had filled his lungs with a full fresh breath. My success in such cases has been to give complete relief from the stammering habit.

REGION BELOW THE DIAPHRAGM

ABDOMINAL AND PELVIC DISORDERS.

In treating such diseases we should remember that the heart delivers the blood to all divisions of the abdomen. It also supplies the brain, thorax, pelvis, limbs and all organs with arterial blood. All divisions of the whole body are supplied by motor nerves and also by the sympathetic ganglia or system of nerves. I think that the major part of the nervous system of the abdomen has for its business the appropriation of the fluids required in the construction and nutrition of the whole body.

When you are consulted on disease of the kidney, womb, bladder, liver, spleen or any organ in the abdomen, and you desire to give a treatment for the relief and return of the organ to normal action, remember the solar plexus has much to do in supplying organs of the abdomen and our first thought should be to find the branch that supplies the organ affected. If we know where that branch is, and proceed accordingly, we will gently pull away the stomach, omentum or any substance covering and making too great pressure on it, or on the solar plexus, aorta or vena cava. A question comes to us. How is the solar plexus nourished? If we go to the great splanchnic I think we will find our question answered.

When you have taken the pressure or constriction off the solar plexus, then you should explore from the semilunar ganglia back through the diaphragm and over the whole splanchnic system. Here you have one of the conductors of nutrition. Here is your work. Begin about the fifth rib and go downward. Without this knowledge our strong treatment is liable to do injury in the place of getting the results hoped for. The object is blood to and from; nerve force to and from. Here you have the advice which I think will guide you in all your questions about diseases of abdominal organs, heart and lungs.

If a person has no idea of the origin and duty of the nerves coming from the solar plexus to the kidney or bladder, he may do great injury. If he is ignorant of the solar plexus, he has no compass to guide him in such diseases as dysentery, constipation, indigestion, enlarged liver or spleen. When he treats such cases, he begins to claw, pull, push and knead the bowels. Then with great force he sends the knee up and down the back and says to the patient, "return in two days and I will give you a stronger treatment if this does not give you relief." The patient has paid him for good work and gets a manifestation of physical strength and ignorance but not value received. To get good results, your head full of anatomy must guide your hands to correctly adjust from the abnormal to the normal with the exactness required for a perfect articulation. Brute force is dangerous. Hands off unless you know your business. Acquaint yourselves with all structures by a deep and continued study of anatomy, because on this foundation you must stand or fall.

HYSTERIA.

Definition.—A disease, mainly of young women, characterized by lack of control over acts and emotions, by morbid self-consciousness, by exaggeration of the effect of sensory impressions, and by simulation of various disorders. Symptoms of the disease are hyperesthesia; pain and tenderness in the region of the ovaries, spine, and head; anesthesia and other sensory disturbances; choking sensations dimness of vision; paralysis; tonic spasms; convulsions; retention of urine; vasomotor disturbances; fever, hallucinations, and catalepsy.

—Dorland.

Definition.—(Hystera, uterus). A neurosis, so called because reputed to have its seat in the uterus (hystera). It generally occurs in paroxysms, the chief characters of which consist in alternate fits of laughing and crying, with a sensation as if a ball—globus hystericus—is ascending from the hypogastrium toward the stomach, chest, and neck, producing a sense of strangulation. There are sometimes loss of consciousness (although the presence of consciousness generally distinguishes it from epilepsy) and convulsions. Hysteria appears to depend upon irregularity of nervous distribution in very impressionable persons, and is not confined to women, well-marked cases being occasionally met with in men. No lesion of the central nervous system has been discovered. During the fit dashing cold water on the face, stimulants applied to the nose or exhibited internally, and antispasmodics form the therapeutical agents. Exercise, tranquility of mind, and agreeable occupations are prophylactics. Chronic paroxysmal cough—hysterical cough—frequently occurs, seeming to be a convulsion of the muscles of the larynx and diaphragm, resembling the cough excited by inhalation of chlorine and other gases.

—Dunglison.

How much time would a traveler spend with a person whom he meets on the road and asks: "My friend, tell me the way to Jerico?" if the man replies to the traveler, "I do not know anything of the road to the city you have named." After telling the traveler that he knew nothing of the road leading to Jerico, of what use would his directions be to the traveler? What traveler would expect to find Jerico by the directions of a man who says, "I am a stranger and cannot give you any of the information you desire?" What traveler would have such little reason as to tarry and spend time with a man who says, "I do not know anything of the country nor the roads leading to the city to which you desire to go?"

The point I have tried to make plain to you is, if all writers acknowledge they do not know the cause producing such disease, why not drop them out and use the compass of reason to find the road that leads to the cause producing such effects. We are at perfect liberty to use our own powers of reason, and hunt for that which has never been found—the cause producing the effect known as hysteria.

Etiology and Examination.—Some writers mix this subject up with epilepsy or chorea, but who among them says, "for cause of convulsions explore the spine above the diaphragm; for cause producing hysteria explore the spine from the diaphragm to the coccyx." Halt at the solar plexus and see if the branches supplying the uterus, the kidneys, the liver and the organs of the abdomen in general are free from any disturbances. I never found a case of hysteria or epilepsy with a perfectly normal spine, ribs, sacrum and coccyx. If we reason as engineers we will generally find that in convulsions the cause lies above the diaphragm and in hysteria in the nerve and blood supply below the diaphragm.

We should care but little for analysis of blood, urine or any fluid passing through the human body when we have a case of epilepsy or hysteria. We know well enough that analysis will show much variation of the quantity, quality and microscopic appearance of the fluids. We know that such conditions do not and cannot appear without a cause; therefore, we should hunt until we find the cause that has produced the nerve disturbance, hysteria, gall-stones, renal calculi and stony deposits of the bladder. They are all effects of some cause. Our business is to find and remove the cause; we can analyze the fluids after recovery. The patient's recovery should be the aim and object of the operator.

As operators we should reason that a further cause is brought about by inhibition of the nerve and blood supply of the maternal organs. This is a result of falls, lifts and strains which push the maternal organs down into the pelvis where they are held in an impacted condition by the colon which in many cases is lying on top of the nerve and blood supply of the uterine system.

Treatment.—With the patient in the knee-chest position, I gently place my hands on the lower part of the abdomen and bring the bowels from the pelvic cavity. This adjustment should be made a few days before and a few days after menstruation. Correct all variations of the coccyx, also any variations of the innominates with the sacrum. Adjust the fifth lumbar with the sacrum and be sure to adjust all lumbar articulations. This treatment has brought results satisfactory to myself and patients.

MENOPAUSE.

Definition.—Natural cessation of the menses, occurring usually between the ages of 45 and 50.

—*Dunglison.*

The uterus has the power to construct itself from an atom to the full form. It has the power to perform such duties as are required of it by Nature. Like a tree it passes through three conditions. The first is the condition of production, or the period of growth from the germ to the full grown uterus or tree of life. This condition lasts from birth until puberty. Then we have the fruit-bearing period or the summer season of the year, which lasts from puberty to the menopause or fall season, when the time for fruit production has passed. Then the leaves of the tree which have filled the place of lungs and purified all substances necessary to the growth of the tree fall off and after a time they appear again and more fruit is produced. Just so it is that the mother produces her fruit, has a resting spell and then produces another child, until because of old age and infirmity the system fails to rally and produce any more fruit.

The period of menopause, or the disappearance of the monthly menses, has a time of preparation lasting two or three years, during which period the system labors to produce this halt in the flow of uterine fluids and many nerve disturbances show themselves, such as mental disturbances, irritability, despondency, etc. The mechanic asks the question, why do these variations from the normal appear? In answer to that question I will say, that had the nerve and blood supply kept the excretory systems up to the normal, normality would have been the result, but the nutrient system of the uterus is worn out and lies down to rest. The tree grows old and older, and death is the result of its labors. During the ten to thirty years in which the uterus has labored, the muscles (and their nerves) that should hold it in place have become exhausted; also the nerve and blood supply to the whole abdominal and pelvic systems have suffered losses in vitality.

What will we do for the suffering woman during the time she passes through the stage known as her menopause, when she is in a condition of nerve irritation that disturbs the whole body? Where is the friction that has produced the stoppage of the excretory system and retained the fluids in the body long enough to ferment and produce those flashes of heat and innumerable aches, pains, etc., that appear in any part of the system as annoyances? These fluids should have been promptly thrown off. As a mechanic I have tried to draw the attention of the mechanical philosopher to the fact that during the days of menopause there is no hope of reproducing a normal child-bearing uterus. Our work is to adjust the body and all the parts that pertain to uterine life from all abnormal conditions which have accumulated from puberty to sterility.

Treatment.—With these facts before us we must explore and adjust all articulations beginning with the head and atlas, and continuing to all joints of the neck, spine and ribs clear through the lumbar to the sacrum and coccyx. Then the innominates and all their articulations with the sacrum, the symphysis pubis, and all the muscles and ligaments of the pelvis, which by childbirth have been pushed too far out or too low down and are producing an irritation of the nerves and muscles at the lower part of the vagina—the coccygeal system of nerves and muscles, the symphysis system, the bulbi vestibuli and the clitoris. Insert two fingers into the vagina, and with the soft parts of the fingers facing the rectum, spread the fingers until there is slight pressure on either side, then pass the fingers from the anterior part of the vaginal opening to the posterior part. Do this in order to free the glands of Bartholin and give freedom and vitality to the pelvic nerve and blood supply. Then fold or push the nymphae inwards and bring all the soft parts that have been strained or misplaced from childbirth back to their natural position in the pelvis. These soft parts may be replaced by placing the patient over the lower end of the table with face downward. Then, without any exposure, push or bring the soft parts from the tuber ischii back into the pelvis. After this is done inhibit over the clitoris to take down or overcome all irritation. Remember that during childbirth the bladder is often drawn down and closes the water ducts from the kidneys to the bladder, and it is our work to put all these soft parts in place. As to washing, curetting, and so on, I have never found any use for them after I adjusted the uterus and brought it above the pelvic floor to its normal position.

Another method; I have my patient while on the treating table lie on her right side; draw her knees up towards her face, to a comfortable position.

Then push all of the muscles of the perineum back to their normal position. This can easily be done with hands on outside of the clothing. No exposure is necessary. This will generally correct the coccyx and all muscles attached.

While the patient is in the knee-chest position gently draw the whole abdominal system up so as to give freedom to the pelvic circulation and to the nerves back to the solar plexus.

GOUT.

Definition.—Gout received its name from (Fr.) goutte, drop, because believed to be produced by a liquid which is distilled drop by drop on the diseased part. Name was first used about 1270. Gout is an inflammation of the fibrous and ligamentous parts of the joints, and is accompanied by an excess of uric acid and deposits of urate of sodium in and around the joints. It generally attacks, first, the great toe, whence it passes to the other smaller joints, producing or being attended with sympathetic phenomena, particularly in the digestive organs; after this it may attack the greater articulations. It is extremely fugitive and variable in recurrence, and may be acquired or hereditary. In the former case it rarely appears before the age of thirty-five; in the latter it is frequently observed earlier. It is often difficult to distinguish it from rheumatism. Pathologically and etiologically the distinction between the affections variously designated gout, rheumatism, rheumatic gout, chronic rheumatism, chronic gout, rheumatoid arthritis, arthritis deformans, etc., has not yet been satisfactorily made. During the paroxysm of gout a burning, lancinating pain is experienced in the affected joint, with tumefaction, tension, and redness. One or more joints may be attacked either at the same time or in succession, and in either case the attack terminates by resolution in a few days. This is acute, inflammatory, or regular arthritis, regular gout, or podagra. At other times pains in the joints exist of more or less acute character, the swelling being without redness. These pains persist, augment, and diminish irregularly without exhibiting intermission, and consequently without having distinct paroxysms. The disease is then called atonic, asthenic, imperfect, or irregular, or chronic gout. It may appear primarily or succeed attacks of regular gout.

Gout may also attack internal organs, when it is called arthritis aberrans or erratica, podagra aberrans, wandering, or misplaced, or anomalous gout. Retrograde or retrocedent, abarticular, extra-articular, flying, recedent, or displaced gout, arthritis or podagra retrocedens, is when it leaves the joints suddenly and attacks some internal organ, as the stomach, intestines, lungs, brain, etc.; the term arthritis uratica has been applied also to gout resulting from abnormal exudations of urates into the articular cavities and the parenchyma of the cartilage, bones, etc., bounding the joints.

Gout is also called, according to the part affected, podagra, gonagra, chiragra, etc. It may be acute, or chronic, and give rise to concretions, arthritic calculi, chiefly composed of urate of sodium, or to nodosities, when it is called arthritis nodosa.   —*Dunglison.*

Etiology.—I have given above the elaborate definition of gout as given by Dunglison. If it is of any benefit to the osteopathic philosopher he can use it. I think that all the symptoms marshalled in the description simply testify to the effects that follow stagnation of the fluids, both nerve and blood, that should supply the muscles, ligaments, bones and the nervous system of the parts affected.

I have observed that most persons suffering with gout, whom I have treated have been merchants or clerks, and those people who are called upon to stand much in an erect position, reaching up with both arms and tip-toeing to place goods up on high shelves. As a mechanic I have reasoned that in this position the upper part of the spine is thrown too far back causing a strain on the lumbar portion which in these cases I have found quite anterior.

Above the lumbar as far up as the eighth dorsal I have found the ribs pulled off and held under, the processes of the vertebrae. I have reasoned that the intercostal nerve and blood supply are perverted from normal action, thus we have stagnation, fermentation and inflammation of the parts through chemical processes acting on the fluids thus detained. This form of straining when followed for a long time produces marked displacement of the eleventh and twelfth ribs on both sides, in many cases bringing them downward with heavy force on to the lumbar muscles, nerves, blood-vessels and the excretory system of the lumbar region. I find also a great deal of thickening about the hip joint.

We are told that gout shows its first work nearly always in the great toe. In all such cases where there was much suffering I have found that this joint was partially and sometimes completely dislocated with the tendon over on the outside of or cramped by the sesamoid bones. I have proven to my satisfaction that the irritation known as gout is an effect following subluxation of that joint. The proof that has guided my conclusions is that when I properly adjusted the big toe and got the tendon in its natural position, soreness left the foot and normal action and ease followed. Hence, I look upon what is called gout as the effect of some abnormal position of the bony structure, brought about by some such strain as is above described. This applies, so far as I have examined, to what is called rich man's gout as well as it does to poor man's gout. In each type I have found these same conditions existing.

Treatment.—My first work in treating patients suffering with gout is to give relief to the great toe by adjusting it and bringing the tendon into its natural position. I generally wrap a handkerchief around the middle of the big toe, very tight so it will not slip, the patient sitting in a chair, the affected foot between my knees. I place my fingers between the great toe and the one next to it with my thumb on the side of the long bone with which the toe articulates. I hold here very firmly while the foot is clamped between my knees, then with my other hand I pull and bend the big toe with considerable force towards the other toe. In doing this I gap the joint and bring the big toe into its proper place. But before I let it go I change my fingers to the under side of the foot and draw the tendons into line between the sesamoid bones. While I have the foot between my knees I adjust all the bones of the foot. In order to do this I generally take the foot in my hands, place the hollow on the inside of the foot against my knee, firmly holding the os calcis in one hand while with the other hand I take hold at the toes and give the foot a few gentle semi-twists and the work is done.

When there is much suffering at the knee as is often the case when the fibula is back or forward and out of its articulation at either end, I take my patient by the ankle while he is still seated and straighten out the leg as I stand on the inner side of it so that I may bring this part against my knee. With my other hand I take firm hold over the head of the fibula. Now with the hand at the ankle I draw the leg out straight, then in order to gap the articulation I raise it a little up and backward and draw head of fibula forward to its place. This is a simple and easy method by which the fibula is adjusted. After this I have my patient take the position on his knees, on the floor, his chest on a stool as is described in detail in the treatment given for lumbago. In giving this part of the treatment be very thorough as it is very effective. Now give special attention to the eleventh and twelfth ribs adjusting them very carefully. Then go on up as far as the eighth dorsal adjusting every variation found in vertebrae or ribs.

I have given you my methods of adjusting the bones in such conditions as are known as gout, rheumatism, neuralgia, and so on and can only hope that the osteopath can comprehend and apply them and gain as large a success as has followed my efforts in giving relief to those suffering from the conditions named.

HEMORRHOIDS.

Definition.—Livid, painful excrescences from the mucous membrane of the rectum or anus, usually attended with discharge of mucous or blood. The most common causes are a sedentary life, accumulation of faeces in the rectum, violent efforts at stool, pregnancy, etc. The precursory symptoms are pains in the loins, stupor of the lower limbs, and uneasiness in the abdomen and rectum, with more, or less gastric, cerebral and general disorder, constituting a hemorrhoidal diathesis. *** To these symptoms follow one or more round, smooth, painful, pulsating erectile tumors around the margin of the anus or within the anus; some bleeding occasionally. Hemorrhoids are sometimes divided into bleeding or open piles and shut or blind piles. They have also been divided into internal or occult and external according to their situation, and into accidental or constitutional. Hemorrhoidal tumors are formed of a close, spongy texture, similar to that surrounding the orifice of the vagina, and, like it, erectile. *** The internal bleeding pile is a soft, red, strawberry-like elevation of the mucous membrane, called a vascular tumor. A leucorrhea analis, or whitish discharge from the anus, sometimes attends ordinary hemorrhoids.

—Dunglison.

Etiology.—I have given you Dunglison's definition which contains about all of the information that the osteopath may expect to obtain from medical literature. The mechanical osteopath who is well versed in the anatomy of this region, its blood supply, its drainage and the functioning processes of the nervous system sees nothing whatever in this definition that is satisfactory or beneficial regarding the cause which has produced this condition.

Constipation following sedentary life is spoken of, but the question arises why is one sedentary person afflicted with this condition while another one just as sedentary is not? On his exploration for cause of this paralytic disturbance of the rectum he goes to the coccyx and in all of the cases he finds it partially dislocated in its articulation with the sacrum, and in many cases a complete separation exists between the two bones. He also goes to the sacrum and finds it tucked in or pushed out enough to separate it from the coccyx.

This condition the osteopath adjusts, and his patient may be expected to get well. He as a mechanic should know that he has found and corrected one cause of hemorrhoids.

Then we explore farther up the spine for the cause of constipation and on careful examination we find the bones of the lumbar region varying from their normal position. We often find imperfect articulation at the fifth lumbar, the spinous process leaning either to the right or to the left, or being too far back or too far forward. We then continue our search upward and find in some cases an imperfect articulation of the first lumbar with the twelfth dorsal vertebra. Also some of the ribs are out of their proper articulations. Going on up the spine we often find imperfect articulation of the fourth, fifth, sixth, seventh and eighth dorsal vertebrae and ribs. We reason that if the ribs are thrown either up or down from the transverse processes, such a condition would obstruct both blood and nerve supply to the spine and ribs as well as to the great splanchnic nerves as they leave the spinal cord; consequently, temporary paralysis or inhibition of the semilunar ganglia of the solar plexus would be the result of such obstruction. When the patient complains of headache, dizziness and tenderness at the union of the neck with the head, then we should carefully explore the neck and know that all joints are in their proper articulation from the occiput to the dorsal.

Treatment.—When I have a case of hemorrhoids or protrusion of the bowels or any such condition to treat, I bring my patient up to the end of the table, place a pillow there and have him lie on it resting his breast and abdomen thereon while his feet are on the floor. At this time and in this position I carefully explore in the region of the coccyx to ascertain whether it is twisted or pushed to the right or left or under the lower part of the sacrum, always leaving the parts covered by some clothing. I never find it necessary to expose a patient in any manner. While I have my patient in this position I place my thumbs, one on each side of the coccyx and push in strongly, using sufficient force on the coccygeal muscles to draw the coccyx down and under. I rotate the coccyx to the right and to the left, then with my right hand while standing at the side of my patient I make sure that I have obtained a good natural condition of the sacrum and the coccyx.

Now I proceed to adjust the spine from the sacrum to the dorsal region, taking every vertebra separately. I do this having my patient take the kneeling position with his chest on a stool about fourteen inches high. Then I grasp his thighs between my knees, holding him firmly while I rotate his body, making a fixed point at each vertebra as I go on up the spine, and make sure that every vertebra is in its normal articulation. Then I adjust the dorsal and the cervical vertebrae, and also the head upon the atlas.

I give the coccygeal treatment once or twice a week if necessary. I never insert my finger into a patient's rectum, to make this adjustment; first, because I think there is no excuse for such an irritation, and second, because we should have some respect and regard for the patient's modesty. I will say for the encouragement of the operator that I have had cases where the bowel would prolapse and protrude from two to four inches and after this method of treatment the rectum went back into the body without any direct local manipulation whatever. Constipation and all abnormalities of the bowels disappear after this treatment.

OBSTETRICS OPERATING WITH INFANTS AND CHILDREN

OBSTETRICS.

(This chapter is not written as a treatise on obstetrics but for the benefit of the young obstetrician in emergency cases.)

Definition.—The art of managing childbirth-cases; that branch of surgery which deals with the management of pregnancy and labor.

—*Dorland.*

Obstetrics is a term used to designate the mechanical manipulation used by an obstetrician in delivering the uterus of the fetal contents when it has finished the work of constructing a human body known as a child.

In studying obstetrics the student should acquaint himself with the normal pelvis and a normal delivery, because more than 90 per cent of all cases are of that kind. Our works on obstetrics seem to lose sight of the normal and hold up the horrors of the abnormal before the young operator. I think it is a mistake to spend so much time in talking and lecturing upon and illustrating with cuts and pictures cases of delivery through a pelvis with the worst possible deformities. It is normal midwifery we want to know and be well skilled in. This you cannot know by a study of the abnormal only. You will likely never find two abnormal conditions presenting the same form of bone or pelvis. If you have a normal condition fixed in your mind you will detect all variations from the normal and be prepared to govern yourself accordingly. If on examination you have an abnormally formed pelvis you will have plenty of time to call counsel and can then be governed by the conclusion.

DEVELOPMENT OF THE FETUS.

Nature has placed all the functions of animal life under laws that are absolute and must be obeyed. Just as long as digestion and assimilation keep in harmony and the mother generates good blood in abundance, the child grows; and by nature the womb is prepared to carry the work of building the body of the child on to completion.

Note the similarity of the stomach and womb. Both receive and pass nutriment to a body for assimilation and growth. When the stomach is overloaded digestion and assimilation stop and sickness begins; then the decaying matter is taken up by the terminal nerves and conveyed to the solar plexus, and the nerves of ejection throw the dying matter out of the stomach. Apply this reasoning to the stomach below, which sickens and unloads its burden. Is this sickness natural and wisely caused? If this is not the philosophy of midwifery, what is?

As soon as a being takes possession of the womb, the commissary of supplies begins to furnish rations of blood for that being, which builds for itself a dwelling-place. The house or child must be built strictly to the letter of the specifications. All the material to be used in the house must be exact in form and of given strength, sufficient to furnish the forces that may be necessary in the future to execute the hard and continued labor of mind and body. Much bone and flesh must be put into its body and some of all elements known to the chemists must be used and wisely blended to give strength.

The manufacturing chief, through the quartermaster, delivers a full supply of all kinds of material for the work. A question is asked: On what road does the quartermaster send the supplies? There is but one system over which the supplies are brought and that is the uterine system of arteries.

When the engine is complete the stay-chains should be cut and let it run out of the shop on an inclined plane. The machinist opens the door of this great manufacturing shop and the engine rolls out by the powers and methods prepared to deliver finished work. The door opens because the lock is taken off by a key that fits and opens it. Muscles that have for so long a time held the door shut stop their resistance, and other muscles by getting sick, convulse with sufficient force to easily push the new engine of life out into open space by natural methods. Be careful that the engine does not deface or tear the door as it comes out.

MORNING-SICKNESS.

When a woman disregards the laws of Nature to such an extent as to over-load the stomach beyond its powers and limits, distending it so that it occupies so much space as to cripple the process of digestion and retain the food, decomposition will set up an irritation of the nerves of the mucous membrane to such an extent as to cause sickness and vomiting. When the nerves of absorption are furnished with material which is not nutritive but destructive and detrimental, the effect of such substances is to cause an irritation of the nerves and they proceed to relieve the system by "unloading."

The stomach is a sac, and when filled to its greatest capacity, it irritates all the surrounding tissues and they in turn irritate the stomach. So naturally, it unloads to get relief. Another vessel similar in size and action is the womb or uterus. It receives nourishment for a being, which nourishment is contained in the blood, and is conveyed to it in the channels commonly known as uterine arteries. This nourishment is taken there to sustain animal life, and is appropriated to the development and growth of the human being.

The placenta in the womb is provided with all the machinery necessary for the preparation of blood to be used in the formation and development of the child. The stomach and the womb receive and distribute nourishment to sustain animal life. Both get sick; both vomit when irritated; they discharge their load by the natural law of "throw up" and "throw down." Note the similarity and the differences and govern yourselves accordingly. The one is the upper stomach that takes coarser material, refines it and keeps the outer man in form and being. The other contains the inner man or child which, when it becomes an irritant, is thrown out by the nerves that govern the muscles of ejection.

At this time the arteries and nerves are active in the development of the fetus, and any disturbance of their normal work is a cause for this sickness. Osseous disturbances by interference with the blood and nerve supply are a very frequent cause of morning-sickness. Often the bowels are filled with dry fecal matter and press upon the uterus, rectum, bladder, blood and lymph vessels, and cause irritation of the nerves of the organs of the abdomen and stop healthy action of all the abdominal viscera. The weight of the womb, the large and small intestines, and the other organs of the abdomen pressing upon the nerves of the pelvis, are causes of morning-sickness in pregnancy. When the normal flow of the fluids that enter into the formation of urine is confused these retained fluids being poisonous affect the solar plexus causing sickness at the stomach, and the vomiting is one way to get such poisons out of the system.

Previous to proceeding with operations to relieve the stomach of this irritable condition we should refresh our minds as to the nerve and blood supply of the uterus and other abdominal organs. Know the nerve supply of the uterus and be familiar with the ovarian and hypogastric plexuses, also the sacral nerves. The blood supply of the uterus comes from the uterine and ovarian arteries, with which the student should be familiar. With the patient in the knee-chest position give free passage of blood and other fluids in the abdomen and remove any impacted condition by placing the hands low down on the abdomen and gently drawing the contents of the pelvis forward toward the umbilicus and upward from the pelvis.

PREPARATION.

A student of midwifery can only learn a few general principles before he gets into the field of experience. Actual contact with labor teaches him that much that he has read is of but little use to him at the bedside. What he needs to know is how to do the things he will have to do after he gets there. He should know the form and size of a woman's pelvis, and how large is the canal through which the child's head will soon come; a normal head cannot come through a pelvis that has been crushed in so much as to bring the pubes within 1½ to 2½ inches of the sacrum. More than 90 per cent of all cases, however, are of a very simple nature.

OBSTETRICIAN'S FIRST DUTIES.

The mother is warned of the approach of her delivery by pains in the back and womb repeated at intervals of one half hour or less, and a physician is called. The first duty of the obstetrician is to carefully examine the bones of the pelvis and spine of the mother, to ascertain if they are normal in shape and position.

First Examination.—Make the examination with the index finger. If there is any doubt about the spine and pelvis being in good condition for the passage of the head, and you find the pelvic deformity enough to prohibit the passage of the head, notify the parties of the danger in the case at once; that there is danger of death to the child and to the mother, but less danger to the mother than to the child; and that as instruments may have to be used in this case, you do not want to take the responsibility alone but wish the counsel of another experienced doctor. The importance of an early examination of the pelvic bones is to give time to be ready for any emergency.

211

Then with the index finger examine the os uteri. If it is found to be opened to the size of a quarter or half dollar, labor has begun. If it is closed and there is only backache, have the patient turn on her right side, and place the hand on the abdomen above the pelvis and gently press or lift the belly up just enough to allow the blood to pass down and up the pelvis and limbs. At this time relax all the nerves of the pelvis, at the pubes.

Second Examination.—Wait a few hours and examine the os again. If still closed and no periodical pains are present, you are safe to leave the case in the hands of the nurse instructing her to send for you when pains return at regular intervals. On your return, explore the os again, and if it is found to open as large as a dime, you are notified that the uterus has begun its work of delivery. Do not place the patient flat on her back because the combined weight of the child, uterus, placenta and fluids, lying on the nerves that control the uterus in delivery disable them so they cannot perform their function properly. Place the patient on her back in a semi-erect position which allows the womb to fall forward and takes pressure away from the nerves. A common chair inverted at the head of the bed so as to make an inclined plane on which the patient's body will rest in a semi-erect position, with a folded quilt and a pillow, provides for very much less uterine and abdominal weight. While in this position the head of the child is easily forced into the pelvis and the perineum is brought back and out of the way of the coming head.

HOW TO PREVENT LACERATION.

Soon you will find in the mouth of the womb an egg-shaped pouch of water which you must not rupture until very late in labor, for fear of stopping the expulsive pains. Remember that while the head is in the fluids of the amniotic sac it turns in the pelvis to suit the easiest passage between the bones.

Now it is your duty to prevent rupture of the perineum. To do this the operator takes a position at the patient's right side, and with the patient in the position above described a slight amount of work with the fingers will prevent any laceration of the perineum. Place the fingers of the left hand firmly over the symphysis and push the soft parts down. With the thumb of the right hand against one of the tuberosities of the ischium and the fingers against the other tuberosity support the perineum with the ulnar border of the hand pressing

212

the tissues strongly against the bones. This allows the stretching of the parts to take place at the sides of the vagina and prevents laceration. If you follow this law of Nature, laceration may occur in one out of a thousand cases, and you will be to blame for that one.

CARE OF CHILD AND CORD.

Now you have conducted the head safely through the pelvis and vagina to the world. You will find the pains stop right short off for about a minute, and that is the time to learn whether the cord is wrapped around the child's neck. If it is found twisted around the neck once or more, you must slip a finger around the neck and loosen the cord, to let blood pass through the cord until the next pain comes, in order to ward off asphyxia of the child.

When the next pain comes place your hand under the back of the child's head and remove the remaining part of the child's body from the mother. Never draw the child too far from the placenta by force as you may tear the cord from the child and cause it to bleed to death. Turning the child on its side remove from the mouth and face all the fluids which might strangle it. Then blow a cold breath on its face and breast to stimulate the lungs to action. When pulsations cease in the cord and the cry of the child shows the lungs are in good action, tie the cord. Beginning at about three inches from the child's belly strip the cord between the thumb and finger toward the child's body in order to remove from it any bowels that may be in it. Then tie the cord with a strong string in two places, one three and the other four inches from the child's body. Cut the cord between the two strings tied around it and exercise care to avoid injuring the other parts with the scissors.

To dress the cord cut a hole the size of your thumb in a doubled piece of cloth five inches long by four wide; cut the hole two inches from one end, run the cord through the hole and fold the cloth over it. Keep the cloth in place by adjusting a belly band over it.

DELIVERY OF THE AFTERBIRTH.

The afterbirth has grown tight to the womb and for nine months has furnished all the blood to build and keep the child alive and growing in the womb. It has done all it can for the child and is now ready to be delivered from the womb. When the child is being expelled from the uterus we very often hear a "cluck" or sound made by the air filling the vacuum in the uterus. When this occurs the air is sufficiently irritating to cause contraction of the uterus on the placenta. Then we have slow delivery of the placenta. Should the uterus contract enough to diminish the size of the os we have retention of the placenta. Sometimes the uterus contracts over the entire placenta as a round ball; at other times it makes a powerful circular contraction around the center or middle of the placenta. In the first case we have a tedious delivery of the placenta because of the general contraction of the whole uterus around it; in the other case we have what is called an hour-glass contraction in which the womb forms a circular band around the placenta.

Many methods have been used to break up the spasmodic action of the uterus and cause it to let go its grasp of the placenta, both in general contraction and in hour-glass contraction. I will give only my experience and the method that has been satisfactory to me. I always work with the view of preventing the closure of the os until the afterbirth is expelled. Nerve terminals having much to do with the irritability of the uterus are located in the clitoris, about the symphysis, and in the region of the neck of the bladder; and as soon as the child is born and breathing easily, to prevent the os from being irritated by the chemical action of the air, I place my left hand flat on the symphysis with the heel of my hand above it and my fingers extending as far down as the urethra and inhibit those nerves of sensation. At the same time I place two fingers of my right hand in the vagina and on the perineum close to the rectum and stretch the muscles downward which produces a contraction of the longitudinal muscles of the uterus. I do this soon after the child is born and before any after-pains. In all my practice I have had no trouble in delivering the placenta with this procedure.

POST-PARTEM HEMORRHAGE.

After the child is delivered, hemorrhage may be produced by retention of the placenta in the womb after its separation, thus preventing the contraction of the uterus sufficiently to close the blood-vessels; by retention of a part of the placenta; by inversion of the uterus.

To relieve the hemorrhage I dip my right hand into the blood and insert it into the womb, and with the back of my fingers straighten out any folds or wrinkles that I find on the inside of the uterus, and remove any part of the placenta that has not been delivered. I retain my hand in the uterus for a few seconds or until I feel the uterus is contracting on it. To start up the contraction I pull the hair or scratch the flesh in the region of the symphysis enough to make an irritation. After withdrawing my hand I push the soft parts all back into the pelvis with my right hand, while with my left on the abdomen I draw the uterus up so as to give free action to the nerve and blood supply to the uterus, and in the pelvis and in that vicinity.

For an abdominal binder I use the mother's shirt, if a good strong one, pulling it down to full length and pinning it on the inside of both thighs to hold it in place. Be careful not to bandage high enough to force the uterus down into the pelvis. To hold the uterus up, a folded towel or cotton pad is placed under the chemise and just above the symphysis, never extending more than two inches above, and secured by two safety pins. A folded towel or cotton pad is placed over the labia to take up the discharge.

DIET.

If the patient's general health is fairly good allow her to tell you what she wants to eat and give it to her. Let her diet be in line with her usual custom. You must remember that she has just left the condition of a full abdomen. Lace her up, fill her up, make her comfortable and leave her for six hours; then change her clothes and bedding. If you stop or interfere with digestion for some hours by giving teas, soups and shadows to eat, your patient will be so weakened that it would be dangerous to give her a hearty meal. For thirty years my practice has been crowned with good success. I have never lost a case in confinement. I have universally told the cook to give her plenty to eat. Do not bother the bowels for two or three days. If the water should fail to pass off even after inhibiting the pubic system of nerves, it may be necessary to use the catheter.

215

TREATMENT OF THE BREASTS.

Caked breasts after childbirth, shortage in the milk supply, sore nipples, or lasting tumors of the breast are seldom found where all ribs, vertebrae and the clavicles are in normal adjustment. When the breast becomes hard after childbirth, or when you find a tumor in either breast it is because the venous system has failed to return the blood supplied by the mammary and intercostal arteries. If the clavicle or upper ribs of the diseased side are producing obstructive pressure on the veins they will not carry off the waste blood and keep the breast in normal condition. The clavicles, and the ribs from the first to the eighth are generally found to be partially dislocated on the sternum or the vertebrae. In all tumefactions of the breast I have found ribs down and under the transverse processes. When you are trying to reduce tumors of the breast remember there are azygos veins, also mammary veins draining the venous blood.

To relieve these conditions I adjust the clavicles and ribs and set free the nerve and blood supply. I have given you several methods by which you can adjust the clavicles and ribs, but I will say that in these cases I usually raise the ribs and free the axillary system while my patient is lying on her back. Grasping the arm I bring it outward and upward strongly until I get it as high or higher than the normal position of the shoulder, and at the same time, with my other hand against the muscles and ribs in the axillary region, I bring strong upward pressure toward the head. I complete the movement by bringing the arm to its normal position at the patient's side with firm upward pressure on it and on the ribs and muscles. For shortage of milk supply treat both sides in this manner then the mammary system will go to work and there will be an abundance of milk.

CARE OF BABES AND CHILDREN.

Crying Babies.

The successful osteopath will be employed very often to treat children of all ages. Many babies only a few days or weeks old cry and continue to cry, baffling the skill of the doctor, nurses and all who would give relief if they could. All family remedies and all the mild remedies of the prescribing physician have been tried but the baby cries all night and all day whether asleep or awake. It is a pitiable condition and so felt by all who see the little sufferer. It was a very nice quiet child for the first week, two weeks, six or more weeks, but all at once it wakes up crying and continues to cry. Without giving any more particulars I will give my experience and success with the little sufferers for the last thirty-five years.

I believe that in washing the child, changing its clothes, etc., it is possible for the mother or nurse, by catching it under the arms and lifting it up not thinking of the force she is applying to the soft and elastic ribs and spine, to draw some little rib out of place far enough for the muscle attached to be put on a strain and hold that rib against another rib and pinch the intercostal nerve. In treating such little fellows I take them up with their breast lying on my breast, and in order to open up the axillary circulation place my hands under their arms with my thumbs up in front of the shoulders. Then with the points of my fingers I feel along to see if any rib is varied from its true position. In some cases I have found the rib pushed back between two processes. I would cover the spine with my hands and gently work the ribs towards me with a little downward tendency toward the end of the rib until the little bump disappeared and the rib was adjusted to its proper place. My success has been almost universally satisfactory to the mother, to the babe and to myself. The child would warm up, take its nourishment and go to sleep and that would be the end of the worry of the mother and the misery of the little sufferer.

If the child has a cough, a sore throat or some enlargement of the tonsils I give it very much the same treatment except that I push the scapulae up and throw the shoulders up a little and back from me in order to let the blood into and out of the neck. The enlargement and the soreness have universally disappeared because the venous blood which was the cause of the swelling could then pass on unobstructed.

There is another cry, this time from the bluish looking children. They jump in their sleep as though frightened. I give them a similar treatment directing my attention more particularly to the left side from the middle of the scapula over the ribs, pretty well down over all the ribs on that side. With a little moving up of the ribs and spinal muscles I take any pressure off of the sixth, seventh and eighth ribs of the left side in order to relieve the diaphragm and the nerves that supply this region. Then I raise the clavicle and free the bones of the upper dorsal and neck to take any pressure off of the pneumogastric nerve. In these I have the same good result.

There is another class who suffer with the colic, or cramping in the region of the stomach and bowels, straining at stool with considerable slimy discharge from the bowels and much griping and pain. In treating this class I commence at the lumbar with an easy movement from the fifth, fourth and third lumbar up to the diaphragm, being always very careful to bring the fifth, fourth and third lumbar far enough forward to be sure they are normal. In this same manner I have succeeded far beyond my hope or expectation in relieving the child of its suffering. With this class of dysentery I generally lay them on their face or side at the end of the spinal treatment and gently draw the belly up a little towards the stomach to free the nerve and blood supply to all the organs of the abdomen.

There is another class that cries every time they are handled showing that they are in much misery in some part of their body. I generally find too much diaper between the legs and one or both hips dislocated and continually on a strain. I would advise the mother to take the child's diaper off and hand the child to me. I would take it and adjust the hips, gently stroking down over the hip and along the leg or thigh, for it does not take much pressure with a child because the socket is not more than an eighth of an inch deep and the capsular and other ligaments of the hip joint are very soft and elastic. Remember this; more cripples are produced by the use of too thick a diaper than people who do not reason from effect to cause have any idea of. Hence, the importance of the caution to be given to mother and nurse.

Hand the child back and in adjusting its clothes if there is any thickness of cloth to be used put it farther up on the buttocks, but use just enough between the legs for cleanliness. Keep the babies out of the bath tub for there is where they are hurt from handling and rubbing them too much. Ask Grandma if she can take a wet cloth and wash the baby and she will say, "yes, I have done it for forty years." One asks how I would feed a baby. I would answer, after having adjusted the baby from head to heels and fixed it so that it can digest its food, then give it the good wholesome food with which the family is familiar. Tell the mother to throw all drugs into the fire and she will get along better with the baby.

BED WETTING.

When a child cannot hold its water it is evident that the nerves from the solar plexus to the bladder are heavily compressed. The ischia are too close together. Your work is to open them out, spread them apart. See that the irritation is taken off of the nerves of the urethra and bladder. With the two hands you can spread one ischium from the other. Pull them apart but do not use any force that is liable to injure the spine. Gently adjust the innominates to the sacrum, and correct all sections of the lumbar and dorsal spine. With gentle pressure in front and above the pubis, draw the bladder or uterus up a little, while in the knee-chest position, then the urine can flow to the bladder. By doing this we can remove the abdominal irritation of the bladder which causes a child to wet the bed. I have used this method of treatment in patients of all ages with the same good results.

INFANTILE CONVULSIONS.

Treatment.—I do nothing during the spasm. After it is entirely over I begin at the eighth dorsal and correct all articulations to the sacrum. Be very particular to bring the third, fourth and fifth lumbar far enough forward to give free passage of nerve and blood supply to the sacral and lower abdominal viscera. Also correct any variations from the sacrum to the occiput but more particularly from the first dorsal to the fifth lumbar. Fill the lower bowels with flour gruel, not starch, in order to take off any irritation that undigested food is producing, because this irritation has much to do, with infantile convulsions. Never fail to fill the lower bowels with gruel once a day until the offensive discharges stop, then stop the use of gruel enemata. For many years I have used this method of treatment. It has been successful and satisfactory to myself and the mother because relief from spasms has generally followed.

ABNORMALITIES OF PENIS.

Definition of Circumcision.—The removal of all or a part of the prepuce, or foreskin.

—Dorland.

For the benefit of the osteopath I will say that he should use great caution and never perform circumcision unless it is necessary. I have found it necessary in many cases but whenever I am consulted, even though the surgeon says circumcision is absolutely necessary, I never give my consent to use the knife until I have explored the region of the union of the symphysis. In a large per cent of cases examined I have found the symphysis pressing upon the nerve and blood supply of the penis close to the neck of the bladder. I believe this is because the ischia are abnormally close together. In many of the cases I have examined I have found this condition.

In some cases the penis is in the erect condition, or is drawn to the right or to the left by pressure in the region of the symphysis. In my opinion the innominates have been strained from their normal articulation and are producing a cramping and shutting off of the nerve and blood fluid and all forces.

Treatment.—Separate the ischia so that no pressure can possibly be left in the region of the neck of the bladder or from there on to the neck of the penis. This will give free passage to the blood and nerve supply to all structures from the bladder to the foreskin. Spread the ischia well apart in all abnormal conditions of the penis. I say use the knife when it is necessary, but I have found but few cases where I thought it necessary to remove the foreskin. During the thirty-five years just passed I have followed this method of giving relief to the abnormal conditions of the penis. Do as I have indicated and you will be surprised at the results. You will always have plenty of time. Do your work well and note the results. The osteopath must never fail to know the producing cause of all effects. He should seek to know the cause, remove it and give Nature a chance to repair.

CROUP.

Definition.—Term variously applied to acute inflammation of the mucous membrane of the larynx alone, or larynx and trachea combined, with production of fibrinous exudation, diminishing the caliber of this portion of the air passages and causing a peculiar cough and breathing characteristic of this disease. The term is often used synonymously with diphtheria, with laryngeal or laryngotracheal symptoms.

—Dunglison.

Etiology.—Croup evidently is the effect of contraction of the muscles of the neck and thorax. This contraction begins with the nerve terminals of the pneumogastric nerve in the air cells of the lungs and continues the spasmodic contraction of all muscles of the neck up to the occiput including the muscles of the larynx, pharynx and trachea producing the spasms as we see them in croup.

We find almost a complete shut-off of both nerve and blood supply between the heart and lungs and the brain, the result of which is asphyxia from the lack of air in the lungs. Not only do we find contraction of the muscles of the thorax but those of the entire length of the spine are in a spasmodic contraction resulting from this atmospheric shock.

Treatment.—We have here in our little patient who is suffering with croup, a human being who is dying for the want of normal nerve and blood supply and its perfect circulation. This is the effect caused by the irritated constrictor nerves that are putting in their powerful and destructive forces and shutting off the normal circulation between the heart, brain, lung and pleurae, which parts must be absolutely normal in action or the result is disease leading to death. This child will die if you do not reproduce normal action of the heart, the lungs and the brain; they are responsible for health and harmony and must be free to perform their part.

In my treatment I begin at the occiput and gently inhibit the sensory system of nerves in this locality. When the patient is a child of six years or younger, I take it on its knees in my lap, its breast against my breast, throw its arms over my shoulders then I begin with a hand on each side of the lumbar

222

vertebrae on and above the sacrum, inhibit the nerves and adjust the vertebrae, treating each and every lumbar vertebra in order to open up and free the kidneys that they may excrete the urine and pass it on to the bladder.

From the first lumbar I proceed on up the spine to the first dorsal, laying my fingers flat and drawing the muscles and ribs outwards from the spine. I am very particular to try to secure good intercostal nerve and blood supply because a constriction here from any cause leaves the sensory nerves of the thoracic organs and those on up to the occiput laboring abnormally under such constriction until the mammary and the intercostal arteries and veins are freed and can perform their duties. I am very careful to adjust all of the cervical vertebrae and draw both clavicles well forward; also I draw forward the upper four ribs (gently with a flat hand on a babe or small child), with the object of letting the blood, as it returns from the head, pass on down without any obstruction by bone or muscle. I give careful attention to the upper dorsal, say from the first to the eighth.

When first called to my little patient I treat him, then stay and let him rest an hour or so and treat him again; in the meantime giving him plenty of fresh air. I make it a practice to be certain to be with the patient and remain from five until nine P. M., because a change of wind at this time may produce an irritation of the sensory nerves which are set in action by changes of temperature such as occur during these hours. When the little fellow breathes easily in a comfortable room and goes to sleep, I go back to my office feeling satisfied that I have done my duty and have relieved the sufferer.

As to home remedies that a mother usually has around, such as mild syrups I never prohibit her giving the child a sup occasionally. If it does no good it will at least do no harm and the mother feels herself to be doing something towards relieving the suffering of her child. When the throat and tonsils are quite sore I tell the mother to have some light soup or mild gruel made tasty so the child will take it. Give the child a little sup or drink often to keep the throat free from the sticky and irritable condition due to the raw surfaces.

RICKETS.

Definition.—A constitutional disease of childhood in which the bones become soft and flexible from retarded ossification, due to deficiency of the earthy salts. The disease is marked by bending and distortion of the bones, under muscular action, by the formation of nodular enlargements on the ends and sides of the bones, by delayed closure of the fontanels, pain in the muscles, sweating of the head, and degeneration of the liver and spleen. There are often nervous affections, feverish ness, convulsions, etc.

—*Dorland.*

Etiology.—After consulting medical, surgical and physiological works for the cause of rickets we are left without an answer. We Simply have a list of effects or symptoms which when placed together are called rickets. When a patient suffering with rickets is brought to me, as a mechanic I begin with this question: was this child delivered with forceps? If the answer is yes, I begin to explore for an abnormal position of the atlas or some of the bones of the neck. In all these cases which have come under my observation I have found defective or imperfect articulation of the atlas with the occiput, while from here down to the sacrum I find the spine pushed right, left, backwards or forwards, which in my opinion is sufficient cause for the obstruction of nutrition to the bony framework and the nerve and blood systems of the entire spinal cord. Without any further ceremony I proceed to treat the child.

Treatment.—I proceed to adjust from the abnormal to the normal all bones of the body from the sacrum to the atlas. I carefully articulate the sacrum with the fifth lumbar, then journeying on up I adjust every articulation of the spine with its facets both above and below and make sure that the ribs articulate naturally with the spine. Then in the cervical region I make sure that every bone is in its normal place, particularly the occiput, at which place I am exceedingly careful with my adjustment because I think the medulla and cerebellum have been confused in their action by partial dislocation of the atlas.

In general practice I give this treatment twice a week for two or three months. I feed the child well on good wholesome food and plenty of it. If the weather is warm enough I am very particular to have the child lie on a rug spread out on the floor in order to keep the spine normally straight. The more the child can wallow on the floor the better. Give the child the advantage of free exercise and plenty of good pure air. I have benefited most of such patients when the case was not too far advanced and some of them became strong, healthy children.

SPINAL REGION

THE NUTRIENT POWER
OF THE NERVOUS SYSTEM OR THE LAW OF
FREEDOM FOR ARTERY AND NERVE.

I think the law of the freedom of the nutrient nervous system is equal if not superior in importance to the law of the free circulation of the blood. We find a nerve fiber, trace it to some locality and there we find a great number of capillary arteries in full action sur rounding a nerve plexus with many branches coming to and going from it. Do these nerves absorb this blood and prepare it to be sent on to be applied in forming muscle and tissue? Another question arises; does all flesh pass through the nerve laboratory previous to being formed into muscle or flesh of any kind?

Let us reason cautiously because if the finale of the atoms of flesh is completed by the nerve system then we see that the two systems, nerve and blood supply, must be kept fully normal or we will fail to cure our patients. Let us remember that no atom of flesh in the body is out of connection with the three nerves motor, nutrient and sensory, and that we should know that all muscles and other parts of the body are formed by and act through this nerve energy. In order to succeed in our profession we must work to establish and maintain normal nerve functioning and that can be done by adjustment of all parts that would hinder in the least any perfect action of the three classes of nerves above named.

As nerve energy is the soul and body of all digestion as far as man knows, we will see the importance of keeping all parts of the frame, every joint, every muscle and all connecting ligaments in perfect position without a twist or strain. Then and not till then we will see perfection in nerve functioning. We will see the nerves drink crude blood fresh from the capillary arteries, refine, finish and apply it to form muscle, nerve, vein, artery, bone, brain and kidney. Thus the importance of some knowledge of the fact that the nerves run the workshops of animal life in all of their mysterious successes.

I am sure that the artery takes blood from the heart for the purpose of depositing it into the womb-like cells of the nervous system in which atoms of living flesh are formed by nerve processes that act to give life, motion and form to organs, muscles and all parts of the body. Surely a species of conception takes place as the arteriole connects with a nerve cell which proceeds to form living atoms of flesh. The artery is only a carrier of blood which gives form and life to muscle building. If so, we are prepared to look well to the per feet freedom of the artery, great and small.

To my mind it is not reasonable that blood is in a condition to take its place as flesh when it enters the artery nor when conveyed to the organs or other parts of the system. It is in a semicrude state while arterial fluid and while it is on its, way through the system. I am of the opinion that the laboratory of the nerves is the place in which the arterial blood goes through the final process and the atoms become qualified to make muscle or flesh of any kind.

CEREBROSPINAL MENINGITIS.

Definition.—Cerebral or cerebrospinal or syncopal typhus, epidemic or typhoid or malignant meningitis, petechial fever, cerebrospinal fever, cerebrospinal arachnitis, sinking typhus, malignant or typhoid meningitis, spotted fever; a generally fatal disease, attended with fever, painful contractions of the muscles of the neck and retraction of the head, headache, vertigo, delirium, coma, pain in the back and limbs, tetanoid phenomena hyperesthesia of the skin, and in certain epidemics by a purpuric eruption, whence the designation spotted fever. It is due to the toxins of Diplococcus intracellularis meningitidis, or Weichselbaum's diplococcus.

—Dunglison.

Description and Etiology.—Cerebrospinal meningitis, its cause, its effects and the treatment are all uncomprehended by the medical world, and are so acknowledged by the very best authors. It prevails sometimes as an epidemic and at other times as an endemic dis ease. Sometimes it will attack only one family in a neighborhood and in some cases four or five members of that family, while in other families only one member is stricken down. With this prelude I will give you the history of my observation as to cause, effect, treatment, cure and mortality.

Cholera prevailed in the United States as an epidemic from 1851 until about 1857, the history of which I have given under the heading of Cholera. About seven years later cerebrospinal meningitis—brain, or spotted fever, as it was then called—made its appearance and began to slaughter people by the hundreds and even by the thousands, according to the prevalent reports of those days. All remedies common to medical knowledge proved failures when administered. Post-mortems were held and all that was ascertained was the effects which that dreadful disease produced on the human system. Such post—mortems showed the brain, its covering membranes and particularly the cerebellum and the whole spinal cord to be in a red gelatinous condition, and a red gelatinous substance was found especially on the inside covering of the meninges. The lungs abounded with such substances, also the heart and the kidneys and the entire glandular system was enveloped in it.

Suppose a man or beast is drowned, will we not see the same identical post mortem conditions? The drowned man is laid out on dry land in the warm atmosphere for several days during which time fermentation begins its work of decomposition and this red gelatinous fluid is found in the brain, the spinal cord, the fascia, the arterial, the venous and the glandular systems. A post-mortem will give you this condition of decomposition in the body of a drowned man just as emphatically as it does on a person who died from the effects of cerebrospinal meningitis which is simply another process of strangulation. This so-called disease prevailed almost as an epidemic in many towns and counties in the eastern part of Kansas, Missouri and other states during the period from 1863 to 1865. My observation was extensive. I have been in large councils of physicians held for my own family and also for others. We tried to ascertain the cause of, the effects of and the remedy for that dread disease. It visited my own home and slew four members of my family in spite of all the council could do to prevent it.

Our conclusion was that to combat this disease by drug medication was useless, for drugs, blisters, opiates, purgatives and so on were all used without avail as four of my family died and we did not know either cause or cure. I have not seen the writings of any author that gave even a very little hope of recovery through medication. I saw in all patients spasmodic or tetanic contractions of all of the muscles, particularly those of the neck, and the nearer to the head the tighter the contraction.

I was so disheartened by the loss of my own children and the realization of the utter inefficiency of all known drug medication that I even refused to go and try to relieve my neighbors' children. I felt that I knew and had the authority for it that the coffin was a certainty for them. But my sympathetic nature yielded to the tears and appeals of the sister of a young man, Mr. Studebaker, who came for me to go to their home a few miles in the country to attend him. I found the young man in a semi-conscious state. His neck and jaw were solidly set by muscular contraction. All of the breathing was through the nose and he was at that time throwing off what I called the deadly froth from the nostrils.

As an experiment, and remembering a previous experience, I poured out a half pint of whisky with the intention of letting him take a sup, but convulsively he grasped the cup with both hands and swallowed all of it. It seemed to me his condition was such that he could not live but a few hours and thinking it could do him no harm I let him drink it. In the course of a half hour he seemed to relax and opened his eyes. Seeing the improvement I poured out something less than the first dose of old fashioned rye whisky and gave it to him. I remained, as I then thought, to see the boy die, but in two hours' time the bladder filled up and on its first action he passed fully three pints of urine. Much to my surprise, inside of four hours consciousness returned. The boy showed no signs of intoxication. Knowing his condition had changed, yet thinking he would surely die I went to my home for the night. I returned the next morning expecting to see crape on the door but behold John was up. All spasmodic action had left the muscles and his neck had lost its rigidity.

The question was asked me "what shall we feed John"? I answered "feed him what he wants." I believe in good plain nutritious food and plenty of it. I am no stickler for dietetics. As my home was four miles away I left orders for the father to report to me at 7 P. M. the boy's condition. The word came that John was to all appearances out of danger which proved to be the truth.

Another neighbor with whom I had some hard feelings, came for me and plead with me to go and see his little eight year old daughter who had brain fever. When I hesitated he broke down, began crying and said "Let by-gones go and come with me and help me save my child." At this I broke down and went off with him, crying also, because his many kind words were not endurable. As I concluded to try the whisky again I took a pint with me and gave the little girl a half a tumbler of it and asked her if it smarted her mouth. She said, "No I do not taste it any more than water." This was the answer of all the patients to whom I gave it, plainly showing a loss of taste.

I staid around the house about two hours and gave the patient a second, but smaller dose. I noticed her neck relax, she breathed easier. She called for the chamber and her bladder acted freely. As this family lived within half a mile of my home I returned at 6 P. M. to see if the girl was dead. I found her much improved and in two or three days she was well, up and free from the dread disease.

The reason I resorted to these experiments with the whisky was the memory of the success I had had several years before with a German patient by the name of slick. He lived at Edgerton, Kansas. He kept a saloon and such drinks as were sold in a new country, whisky, wine and brandy. This man was a patient of Dr. Addy who had called me in council because there had died in this neighborhood some fifteen or twenty patients who had suffered in a similar manner. I told the doctor that I would try an experiment on this Dutchman. According to all indications and to every symptom we had both concluded that death was inevitable in at least a very few hours. So taking a large table tumbler I filled it with brandy and took it to the patient as he sat propped up in a chair. He took hold of the glass with both hands and I could not get it away until he drank every drop of it.

This was a case of cerebrospinal meningitis. The patient had heavy congestion of the brain and also of the lungs with exhausting sweats. We thought his life was limited to hours, not days. The doctor and I walked out doors. He said to me "by——Dr. Still, I expect that tumblerful of brandy will do him up." We staid around an hour or two. The exhausting sweats stopped, rationality appeared, the lungs seemed to breathe easier; there was no appearance of intoxication. As I lived ten miles away I promised to return the next day which I did, and in place of finding a dead man I found one entirely relieved and his wife was busy picking the feathers from a scalded hen for his dinner. I reasoned that to keep drinks away from a Dutch man, an Irishman or one who is in the habit of drinking is poor policy, and as this disease, cerebrospinal meningitis, was prevalent and Dr. Addy's practice and skill was considered equal to any in the country, the success in this case resulted in his having many others to treat even though he had lost some fifteen or twenty prior to this one. I saw him occasionally for a year or so and he said he had lost no more such cases but had "brandied" all.

The object was to fill the body with enough alcohol to stop fermentation, which fermentation I believe was the cause of the irritation, contraction and spasms resulting in death. At this time I did not reason that the spasmodic contraction and the stoppage of the blood to and from the brain was the cause that produced these effects resulting in death from cerebrospinal meningitis. But since reasoning as a mechanic I see that such a contraction in the neck between the heart and the brain will leave the blood in an inactive condition and will retain it long enough for decomposition to take place in all organs of the system, and the patient will die from the effects of dead blood the result of stagnation due to obstruction of nerve and blood circulation.

I have given the osteopath the history of these cases of cerebrospinal meningitis and the results that I obtained in the early pioneer days with the use of brandy and whisky, not as a prescription to go by but because this fact was the pointer which led me to philosophize as a mechanic and find the cause of death. I think death in these cases results from contraction caused by irritation which I think began at the lungs after in haling poisonous atmosphere from some decomposing substances in the immediate neighborhood close to the house. This I found to be the case usually. In the case of my own family I found floating on top of the water in our well the bones and feathers of a dead hen, the flesh of which had decomposed and been taken up by the water and drunk by the family. One daughter, myself and our colored man drank strong coffee three times a day while the four children who died did not use it at all. I think the coffee neutralized the effects of the putrid poison that was in the water rendering its effects harmless as neither this daughter, the colored man nor myself were attacked by the disease.

Treatment.—I want to say to the doctor, the mechanic of osteopathy in whose hands and judgment a human life is placed, get it out of this whirlpool of death known as cerebrospinal meningitis. You are now dealing with an engine. You are inspecting one that for some cause is out of running order and on you rests the responsibility of finding and removing the cause of this deadly friction producing these contractions, spasms and death. If you comprehend your business as an engineer you will spend no time analyzing the steam or the tar and the worn out grease that comes out of the axles or off the piston rods, to see what is the matter with the engine. If you can honestly fill the place of a human engineer you will know whether the furnace is open or is stuck together with slimy cinders, and will open it with the shovel of reason. If your furnace is all right, the steam chest and all parts of the engine in good order, all but the escape pipe, you will know this fact or you do not know enough of an engine to be trusted with its management.

I have given you my experience and experiments and practical knowledge of this disease. I have tried to explain and emphasize that the escape pipe or valve is shut off, is out of order so that every structure that unites the neck and the head has undergone a spasmodic tightening and this is the condition that prevents the blood from passing either up or down and is the effect that accompanies this disease. Now we have only to reason back one step to know that poisonous gases or very cold chilly winds inhaled into the lungs will set up a kind of fermentation in the fluids coming to and from the lungs which produces a very high degree of nervous sensation such as always precedes lockjaw or any other spasmodic contraction of the human body at any point or place in the entire system. Our business is to open the steam pipes through which the arterial blood is driven to the brain, and the veins with their valves which drain the blood from the brain and spinal cord.

I always begin this treatment with the patient on his back. I get up at the head of the bed or treating table and carefully inhibit all nerves in the region of the back of the neck and its union with the head. While in this position I want to open out the axilla and get normal blood circulation in it, so with my right hand I take the patient's right wrist and pull the arm out while with my left laid flat I gently draw the axilla and its muscles well out from the body and up. The object of this is to know that I have prepared for both axillary and subscapular blood and nerve supply. Then take the left arm and side through the same process. Do not use any roughness with the points of your fingers but have as your object to secure axillary freedom and know that your entire axillary region is in good condition before you leave it.

Now while we stand at the head of the patient, we hold gently with the flat of our fingers placed firmly between the third cervical and the occiput. Use no wriggling or twisting of the neck, but hold gently and firmly so as to inhibit for a short time the posterior occipital nerves which are really very sensitive and have much to do with the spasmodic contractions and the crowding of the muscles and ligaments and the impingement of the pneumogastric nerves. This contracture is an absolute prohibitor of the return of venous blood in all cases of cerebrospinal meningitis and this spasmodic condition must be removed or taken off.

I correct the clavicles at both ends. I spread the shoulders while I am standing at the side of the bed. Leaving the patient's arms at his side I place the hollow of my hands on the point and upper part of each shoulder, then with considerable force I bear down and Spread the shoulders out being careful to bring both ends of the clavicles to their normal positions because a stagnation due to a misplacement in this region would obstruct the venous blood in its return to the innominate vein which unobstructed return is absolutely demanded. Now we must proceed to adjust the ribs and all of the vertebrae

234

from the sacrum on up to the occiput, and when you have done that, proceed with the flat of your hands, starting at the symphysis pubis and gently open up the ureters from the neck of the bladder on up to the kidneys. Take off all pressure from solar plexus, free the renal and pneumogastric systems.

In reference to diet, nothing is either desired or eaten by these patients during the severe shock. When my patient is relieved sufficiently to want to eat, it has been my rule and method to let them eat any easily digested food. As to beds and room, my patient's comfort is to be considered. I invariably leave the arrangement of both these matters to the family in whose house the patient is. My object centralizes on doing such work as will relieve the patient and get him out of the condition that contraction of muscles has produced, and my process of getting that relief I have tried to make plain to you. Consult the blood and nerve supply to and from the brain and govern yourself accordingly.

LOCOMOTOR ATAXIA.

Definition.—Tabes dorsalis; posterior spinal sclerosis a chronic morbid condition described by Duchenne of Boulogne, prominent symptom of which is loss of power to coordinate voluntary movements, with lightning-like pains in the back, viscera, and lower extremities; the tendon reflexes are lessened or obliterated, and disturbances and irregularities of sensory manifestations occur, together with trophic disturbances in the joints. The lesion is a sclerosis of the posterior root-zones of the spinal cord. The affection occurs in middle age or later, and is generally regarded as parasyphilitic in origin.

—Dunglison.

Etiology.—After perusing many of the latest medical authors on this subject we find that all they have done so far is to marshall, line up and present to the anxious reader the effect of some unknown cause. They tell us that the white man is subject to this disease and the negro is immune; also that syphilis is a cause of the disease. If this be true and syphilis is the cause of locomotor ataxia, why does the negro not suffer with it? A large per cent of the colored people have syphilis but do not have locomotor ataxia. A much smaller per cent of white folks have syphilis and they carry the burdens and tortures accompanying locomotor ataxia. A very great number of white persons have locomotor ataxia yet never have had syphilis in any form. Here we drop medical therapeutics and practice because they have acknowledged they know but little of cause or cure of locomotor ataxia. Let us hunt for a cause that a philosopher would accept, and if we fail in our search let us own our ignorance and join the hosts that have hunted and failed to report anything that gives light on this subject.

Allopathy and homeopathy have been very liberal in administering mercury in some form as a remedy for gonorrhea, syphilis, bilious fever, chills and fever, typhoid and summer complaint. Mercurial ointment has been freely used for skin eruptions, ulcers and so on without limit, even to the use of red precipitate of mercury as a cure for barber's itch. They administer mercury without stint or reason until the system takes up and retains enough mercury to destroy the normality of the dental system of nerves, and the blood supply of the upper and under jaws. It robs the entire nutrient system of its nerve and blood supply; it weakens all joints of the spine and limbs with all of the muscles and membranes that belong to the system of articulation and motion.

The "Pill Doctor" says, "Dr. Osteopath you have not told us why the negro is immune and the white man is subject to locomotor ataxia." I will ask why it is that we seldom find a colored man afflicted with locomotor ataxia, and that when we do we also find that he has had a mechanical injury of his spine. Why is it that a negro can take any quantity of mercury without producing salivation? Why is it that a white man cannot use mercury in any form without producing ptyalism, or salivation? I will ask the mercury doctor what the photographer says of the power of light to produce precipitation on mercury and the power of darkness to prevent it? A photographer is very careful to keep all sensitive plates in the dark until he wishes to produce a picture. Will the sun's rays pass through the white man's skin and deposit mercury close to the bone? Is the negro's black skin penetrated by the rays of sunlight? If not, mercury administered to a negro fails to be precipitated, for his skin acts as a dark room. I reason that the white man's skin does not prevent the rays of light from coming in contact with the mercury in his system and that the mercury is driven to the bones and the continuous action of light on the mercury produces the poisonous action known as salivation. The white man who has mercurial treatment to the degree of salivation is liable to have shaking palsy, locomotor ataxia and general atrophy of the nervous system of spine and limbs. My opinion as a chemist, mechanic and philosopher is that all this bugaboo about syphilis being the cause of locomotor ataxia is without a shadow of reason that could be accepted by any man who reasons from effect to cause. To me, locomotor ataxia in most cases is the effect of mercury and should be treated accordingly.

Treatment.—Believing this disease comes properly under the head of mercurial poisoning and as mercury does not go through the chemical action to precipitate without the aid of light, we know why the negro is immune to the effects of mercury. The inside of his dark skin acts as the dark room of the photographer who depends wholly upon the action of light to produce the effects of light and shadow. He knows that no change will take place in sensitive paper if kept in darkness, but the admission of light produces precipitation immediately and a picture is the effect. Though the body is filled with mercury it may pass off, or may stay leaving such bad effects as rheumatism, locomotor ataxia, etc. The white man's skin offers no resistance to the action of the rays of light from the sun on mercury in his body whether it is given by mouth or absorbed when applied to the skin.

Your fight in combating this disease is to thwart the chemical action of precipitated mercury. As mercury has a greater affinity for red clay (taken from the kind of clay known as cinnabar) than for human flesh we will treat the disease both internally and externally. Make a preparation of common red clay as follows: Take a shovel full of red clay in a vessel and mix it with water until the solution is muddy. Allow the sand and gravel to settle to the bottom then pour off the muddy water into a pan. Repeat this procedure until a dissolution of the greater part of the clay takes place. Leave the pan in open air until you have a precipitation of the clay leaving the water clear on the top. Pour off the clear water leaving the clay in the bottom of the pan to dry out and become a cake. Now it is ready for use and not unpleasant to the taste. If the cake is one half inch thick when dry have your patient eat as much as a two-inch square of this cake before each meal for two days. Then stop one day and repeat the doses morning, noon and night. Be sure to drink plenty of water in order to keep the clay moist and soft to prevent its caking in the bowels. Should it cake in the lower bowels enough to produce constipation, soften by injections of water. Then make a clay poultice a foot wide and an inch thick for the entire length of the spine and extending below the hip joints. Spread the poultice on one edge of a yard of domestic and fold the remaining part over the clay to protect the back and clothes from being soiled. Have the poultice reasonably soft and warm to aid secretion. Use it once or twice a week.

When the sunlight strikes the feces they will be very dark which proves that the mercury is leaving the body. It is being carried off with the clay which is used to take the place of cinnabar in which mercury is found in its native state. After this, osteopathic treatment is all that is necessary. After the first week the osteopath will begin his manipulation of the spine and hip joints which he will find in abnormal condition. These patients have a partial or complete dislocation of the spine and hip joints which should be adjusted at once. Then

238

their suffering gives place to rest. A great many locomotor patients, in fact all that I have treated, have by contracture had the femur pulled upward and backward out of the acetabulum. The spine is very irregular in its articulation from the fourth dorsal to the sacrum and coccyx. I have succeeded in giving relief and ease to all cases with much improvement in locomotion. I promise nothing, but do the best I can to free the patient from the effects of mercury which I think is the chief cause of this malady.

NEURASTHENIA.

Definition.—Nervous prostration; depression due to the exhaustion of nerve-energy. The name for a group of symptoms resulting from some functional disorder of the nervous system with severe depression of the vital forces. It is usually due to prolonged and excessive expenditure of energy, and is marked by tendency to fatigue, lack of energy, pain in the back, loss of memory, insomnia, constipation, loss of appetite, etc.

—*Dorland.*

Etiology.—In exploring for over thirty years for the cause of nerve debility, nerve prostration, hysteria and all this class of disturbed nerve conditions, I have found the cause of much of it in the impoverished condition of the whole sympathetic system from the atlas to the coccyx. It seems to have lost the power to execute the function of supplying the nervous system with nourishment.

In all cases of hysteria, sick headache and all other conditions along the line of this whole list of nerve disturbances I find much variation from a truly normal spine beginning my work with the coccyx and ending it with the atlas. I say that I never have found a single case suffering under any of these conditions with a truly normal articulation of the head, neck, dorsal, lumbar, sacrum and the coccyx. Vertebrae are strained, ribs are off their articulations and cutting off the supply of nourishment to the nervous system. Thus the effect which we see and which is known as nervous prostration, excitement and on to mania.

Treatment.—In my treatment of these patients I confine my explorations for cause to the bones of the spine and ribs. With your knowledge of anatomy I will say we must adjust all bones of the spine and their rib articulations and see that they remain in their natural positions, allowing perfect freedom of all blood vessels as well as all of the nerves. When this work is well done, a treatment once or twice each week is enough. Reasonable exercise, wholesome diet, cheerful company, freedom from all drugs. By working after this plan you may expect good results. This has been my method and it has proven satisfactory not only to myself but also to my patients.

NEURALGIA.

Definition.—Generic name for a very acute, exacerbating or intermitting, throbbing pain, which follows the course of a nerve, extends to its ramifications, and seems, therefore, to be seated in the nerve. It may be due to a variety of causes, local (pressure), central (brain or cord disease), or systemic (diabetes, malaria, syphilis, etc.). According to their seat the principal neuralgiae have been distinguished by various names.

—Dunglison.

Etiology.—I have quoted Dunglison's definition of neuralgia. He and other medical writers give about the same description of this condition of the nerves. I will not undertake to define it any further than to say that all aches and pains are simply manifestations or proofs of nerve disturbance which journeys on with its processes to unbearable suffering. For instance tooth ache is neuralgia. Headache, the suffering in rheumatism, lumbago, sciatica and on through the list, make us know through the sensory nervous system that the cause is abnormal nerve functioning. This crying of nerves or suffering shows to me that the supply of nutrition to the nerve system is diminished or impure. In all the conditions that I have listed I find the normal supply of nerve fluids that should come from the brain is changed in either quantity or quality. Thus the supply of nutritious nerve fluid to the system is diminished, the result of which is the nerve misery experienced, which misery is a cry for food, and the nerve will cry until food comes, as life's palliative and consoler.

I reason that in all cases of neuralgic suffering of the head, spine, limbs, or any organ or part of the body, the part is laboring under obstructed nerve and blood supply which when normal tolerates no misery. For instance, a tooth receives its arterial blood supply, its venous drainage is shut off, congestion, stagnation, fermentation, inflammation, is the result. Thus we may have neuralgia when the nerve and blood supply are not normal from any cause whatsoever. Outside of surgical injuries, we must look for the cause of such confusion in the lack of perfect nerve and blood circulation. I have proven to my satisfaction that this is true in toothache, in tic douloureux, headache, rheumatism of shoulders, of the spine, sciatica, lumbago and all parts of the body where rheumatic or neuralgic suffering is located.

From my observation in all continued or periodic headaches I have found the shut-off in the bones of the neck at their union with the head and in the other joints as far down as the fourth dorsal and even as far as the lumbar, sacrum and coccyx. I have found abnormal positions of both bone and muscle resulting in the production of such effects. I think this is true because when I have a case of tic douloureux or facial neuralgia and have adjusted the inferior maxilla, the atlas, the axis and on to the fourth dorsal, and also the clavicles, the misery disappears. Toothache disappears in the majority of cases, but when the tooth is much decayed or there is much ulceration, I turn such patients over to the dentist. When I find neuralgia in the shoulders, which goes with all rheumatic conditions, I prove this to be an effect by the good results that follow the treatment and adjustment. In giving the treatment I will say a word for each of several neuralgic conditions.

TREATMENT.

Headache.—For continued or periodic headaches I begin in every case at the occiput by laying my fingers flat on the back of the neck over the occipital nerves. Here I bring a gentle and firm pressure for a few minutes during which time I find the muscles relaxing under my fingers on both sides of the neck from the base of the skull to the fifth cervical vertebra. After this inhibition I place my fingers on the transverse processes of the atlas, axis and other upper cervical vertebrae. While doing this I generally press on the top of the patient's head with my breast bringing the pressure downward in the neck towards the body. This loosens the neck. Then I proceed to articulate the facets of all of the joints of the neck beginning with the atlas. After this is done without any twisting or wringing of the neck, which I think is not necessary, I generally stretch the neck up a little giving a slight motion to the right and left holding my fingers on any bone that is out of position. This the osteopath knows how to do.

For this grade of headache I continue this process while I am in front of my patient. Then adjust the clavicles at both ends and particularly at the scapular end and open up the axillary circulation thoroughly, both for the nerve and blood supply. When there is any tenderness in the region of the lumbar I proceed to examine it and make a correct articulation of the fifth lumbar with the sacrum; then travel on up and correct any variation from the normal that I find between the fifth lumbar and the occiput. I do this because I want good nerve and blood supply to the renal system as well as the entire excretory system which must be brought to and left in a perfectly normal condition.

Stiff Neck.—Often people get up in the morning with a stiff neck, a condition which I have generally relieved by standing on the side opposite the one affected and placing the flat of my hand so as to cover the lower part of the neck and one or two of the upper ribs. I bear down gently and strongly with the hand that is on the lower part of the neck, and, while holding firmly, push the head from me with the other hand, then move the head backwards, forwards and towards the hand that is on the ribs and muscles.

Tic Douloureux or Facial Neuralgia.—In all cases that I have examined and treated, I have proven to my satisfaction that this suffering is caused by a shut off of the facial nerve and blood supply on that side of the face in which this periodic misery appears. This shut-off is made by a strained or dislocated inferior maxilla. I place my hand behind and on the angle of my patient's under jaw with a firm hold, then ask the patient to open his mouth. At this time I place my other hand on his chin and bring it forward and down with a firm rotary motion which movement when done properly returns the inferior maxilla to its normal position. It has possibly been thrown out when having a tooth extracted, or by other strains or jars, which have slipped that and often some of the bones of the neck from their normal articulations and have produced a shut-off of the normal nerve and blood supply to the trifacial nerve. I now wrap a handkerchief around my thumb and place it in the mouth as far back on the jaw as the wisdom teeth. I place my other hand on the side of the head, then with my thumb I press the jaw down giving it a little transverse motion.

In every case of tic douloureux which I have had for thirty-five years, I have succeeded in giving entire relief with one or two exceptions, and those were patients who had undergone surgical operations having some of the nerves cut away. I am satisfied the cause of tic douloureux is pressure of the under jaw and upper bones of the neck on the trifacial nerve thus cutting off its supply at that point; and I have given relief to many patients whose trifacial nerves had been operated on by the knife of the surgeon, which operation I know to be wholly unnecessary in any case of tic douloureux. I have given the relief but the distortion or appearance of the face continued as the surgeon left it. I think all cases of tic douloureux can be successfully treated and cured by a skilled osteopath.

Neuralgia or Rheumatism of Shoulder.—The same cause—starved nerves and poor blood supply—is responsible for the neuralgic suffering of the shoulder generally called rheumatism. I bring both clavicles to their normal articulations at both ends. In a large per cent of neuralgic suffering of the shoulder, whether there be swelling or not, I find the outer end of the clavicle pushed too far back. I place my patient on a stool or chair and bring the arm out at right angles, and if there is much tenderness I put my knee under the arm in the axilla, my foot resting on the chair beside the patient. I bring the arm down over my knee and swing it backwards and forwards, then bring it right up and—across the face. I am very particular about making sure of the normal position of the clavicles without which we cannot expect freedom from misery in the region of the shoulder. Be sure you are right before you stop. Other methods are just as good. Our object should be to adjust the bones regardless of any special method.

Lumbago.—In treating lumbago, I place my patient's breast on a stool not more than twelve or fourteen inches high and bring his legs at right angles to his body so that his back forms a bench. While in this position I come up behind him, spread my knees far enough apart to get his hips between them. I then draw my knees strongly against his hips. At this time I place my thumbs on the transverse processes of each lumbar vertebra, beginning with the fifth, then with my knees I give a twisting motion to the lumbar part of his body, then move my thumbs up to another joint and so on up to the eighth dorsal, carefully adjusting each joint. You will soon see that the lumbar is easily moved to the right or left while in this position. This method is easy both on the operator and patient. Repeat this treatment daily until relief is given to the entire lumbar system. My success in applying this treatment in cases of lumbago has been followed by a normal and healthy lumbar region. Any other method is just as good if it does the work.

SCIATICA.

Definition.—A painful inflammation of the sciatic nerve, usually a neuritis. It is attended with paresthesia of the thigh and leg, tenderness along the course of the nerve, and sometimes by wasting of the calf muscles. The pain is constant, but subject to exacerbations. The disease usually attacks persons of middle age.

—Dorland.

Definition.—Neuralgia of the sciatic nerve.

—Dunglison.

Etiology.—Dunglison's definition of sciatica is very short and right to the point. He does not give the cause neither does any author whom I have consulted say anything that is satisfactory regarding the cause which produces this condition.

For the benefit of the osteopath I will illustrate my mechanical reasonings by relating an accident which befell me in 1858. While riding very fast through the prairie grass my horse stumbled and fell flat on his side with one of my thighs and legs under him. With the other foot I pushed the horse off of my leg, got up, mounted him and went on my journey. A few days later I began to feel sore, with back-ache and suffering in the region of the lumbar and hip joint. I never thought for a minute that I had received a dislocation of the hip by the crushing force of the falling horse. I was confined to my bed for two or three months with great suffering and misery in the region described, with fever of my whole body, much headache and restlessness. After some months the fever left me and then I did not suffer so much in my back and hip in the region of the sciatic system. I got around and out and was able to ride horseback and resume my practice. A Mr. Davidson came for me to treat his sick boy, and while riding up hill by his side his unshod horse gave a quick jump, whirled, and kicked at me. I saw the hoof coming and jerked my knee up to get it out of the way, but the foot came high enough to hit me with great force on the knee, driving it back toward the acetabulum. I expected another three months' confinement in bed to follow that kick, but to my surprise when I got off of the horse I felt no sciatic misery either of the spine or limb at that time nor afterwards.

With me this settled all theories regarding the cause of my suffering as well as that of the tens of thousands of other persons who have by falls, kicks, jolts, jars or strains of various kinds had the head of the thigh bone knocked up and out of its socket. Since that time I think I can safely say that I have treated hundreds of cases of sciatic neuralgia, sciatica, or rheumatism (I don't care what you call it) but I want to tell you that as to the cause of it I have invariably found either complete or partial dislocation of the femur from its natural position in the acetabulum and that every one of these cases was not only relieved but after my treatment they got well and went about their business. I have found that very few physicians or surgeons make this slipping out and up of the head of this bone from its socket a foundation to reason from, and therefore they do not give relief to the sufferer by adjusting the hip, the sacrum, the innominate, the bones of the lumbar region or the fibula. This would give freedom to the whole sciatic nerve system from the lumbar region down to the toes.

Treatment.—I have my patient stand at the end of the treating table over the end of which I put a pillow so as not to hurt the patient, and then have him lie down with only the abdomen and chest resting on the table. I stand between his feet with my side toward his body. I then take his foot in my outer hand and place my inner knee into his popliteal space and fix the other hand over the region of the acetabulum and trochanter major. With my knee I press down so as to bring the thigh bone towards the socket. While I hold my knee firmly in the space, I move the leg and foot crossways (to and from the leg on which I am standing) with a gentle movement, and work in the region of the hip joint, gently and firmly. As a result, the tangled condition of the muscles disappears and the hip bone takes its place. While in this position I place my thumb along on the sacrum beginning at the fifth nerve, and continue on up, all the while moving the leg to and from me until I have the sacrum and lower spine in normal condition. This is one of the methods which I use.

Another is to have my patient lying on the table on his back with the legs spread out. I sit on the edge of the table with my thigh well up in his crotch. I then take hold of the patient's leg and with a slight twisting motion I draw the thigh down towards the socket and hold it with my fingers while I flex the patient's knee and bring it in an easy position to get my breast against it. Then I bear down with my breast and rotate the leg outward and inward a few times, then I straighten the leg out across my thigh and twist the foot a little. By this method I have adjusted a great many hips.

Another method I sometimes use is to seat my patient on an ordinary chair with his well side up against the wall. I get down on my knees, place my thumb, on the under side of the trochanter major, my fingers on the anterior surface of the ilium. While in this position I take the patient's foot in my other hand at the ankle. I bend the knee until I can get my chin over against it and in this position I bring the ankle around to my left, if I am adjusting a left hip. Then I throw this thigh across the patient's right knee and make a strong pull down sat the left ankle with the object in view of straightening out the gluteal muscles and capsular ligament. Then I bring the leg off, straighten it out, tell the patient to get up and stamp his heel on the floor. By this method I have successfully adjusted dislocations of the hip, I can safely say hundreds of them.

Now I have given you three methods. I could give you several more but I think this is enough to give you a start ln adjusting dislocations of hips. When there is ankylosis, ulceration or tuberculosis about the joint I treat such cases as a surgeon should.

RHEUMATISM.

Definition.—Rheumatism is a word commonly used to denote a variety of clinical states, the underlying cause of which is supposed to be essentially the same. The disease may attack joints, muscles, or fibrous or serous structures; hence the terms muscular, articular, synovial, cardiac, cerebral, etc. It may be acute, subacute, or chronic in its course and duration. It is characterized subjectively by pain chiefly, which may be severe, lancinating, shifting, or dull and boring, according to the variety of the disease and to the structures involved. Objectively there may be fever, local red ness, and swelling when acute, or no perceptible change in the affected part, or in certain cases great deformity may result from inflammatory changes with secondary contraction and disability. The morbid anatomy and etiology of rheumatism remain doubtful. The causes commonly ascribed are the presence of lactic acid, uric acid, or excess of fibrin in the blood, cold and micro-organisms.

—Dunglison.

Rheumatism is a condition with which the whole world is familiar. There is swelling, soreness of joints in some one part or in the entire body, and locomotion becomes very painful as all persons of any experience or observation well know. Every student of anatomy knows we have a brain with its system of nerves; also arterial, venous and lymphatic systems. When these systems and every articulation of the bony system are in natural working order, ease, comfort and health are the effects.

We get up some morning with soreness and aching in the back of the head, the back of the neck and down along the course of the nerves which should supply the arm and its joints—soreness all the way. Then we travel on down through the spinal cord to where the nerves branch out to supply the lower limbs and here is also soreness and tenderness. Accompanying this headache and soreness there is much or little fever and also a laborious action of the heart.

Etiology.—I have long since been satisfied that all this so-called rheumatic suffering comes from the chemical action of poisonous fluids that should have been normally excreted from the system. I think it is an effect which is the result of impure compounds carried to and deposited in the vicinity of the joints of any part of the body. Bone adjustment according to this philosophy has almost universally given ease and has restored the parts to their original normal condition.

I am satisfied that the difference between rheumatism and neuralgia is that in the former there is an irritation from fermentation of the surrounding fluids with the consequent suffering; while in the latter we have an effect of a starved condition of the nervous system, or of some of the nerves being minus a full supply of nerve fluid, which is followed by the misery of starvation. When we remove the obstructing cause we have the proof of this reasoning because normal functioning is the result in a very great majority of cases of so-called neuralgia.

When any part of the body receives a jolt by a fall, a mental or physical shock or a wound, many kinds of abnormal compounds and fluids are produced, confused, brought together and circulate in the system. If these abnormal fluids are not returned on time but are de posited in the membranes, congestion, fermentation or decomposition of the impure chemical' compound follows.

To illustrate what a shock or injury can produce, I will say that when a boy I went to market with a basket of eggs. In this basket I carried chicken, goose, turkey, guinea, snake, buzzard, eagle, blue bird and grasshopper eggs. I was carrying the basket on my head and when I came to the grocery store I stumbled and fell breaking every egg in the basket. I scraped this conglomerate mess of eggs or glands into a bucket and watched it for a number of days with a powerful microscope. I found various changes taking place in my bucket. I was at a loss to know what to call the process when an old darkey spoke up and said, "I's gwine ter tell yo in sho't what am de 'formance in de bucket. It am nuthin mo' o' less dan rumaticks. It am de effect of bringin de wrong kinds togedder in de bucket an' dat's all der am to it." He said "de doctor say 'rumatoed' an' 'arkitis' an' 'osmofus' an' he keeps 'is mouf gwine 'bout all dese tings. He say 'take dem drops' an' 'take dese drops'; 'jump inter hot water an' jump out'."

This is a rough illustration, but it is a fact that a blow on the head, abdomen, shoulder, hip or foot can produce a shock of the whole nervous system and the effect would be to stop the normal action of the kidney, brain, heart, lung and lymphatics. It will also affect the normal blood circulation, and stagnation, congestion, fermentation, and the production of a poisonous fluid are the results.

When venous blood has been obstructed and retained in the region of the spinal cord and of the cerebellum by impingement or muscle contractures operating to hold the upper cervical bones out from their normal positions, we have a condition that will result in rheumatism. To stop the return of blood from above the articulation of the atlas with the occiput until stagnation sets up in the venous blood will result in heat and inflammation. Constriction and stoppage of blood at this place long enough will form poisonous compounds that take the place of the healthy nerve fluid which should come from the brain. This poisonous fluid taken up by the pneumogastric and cardiac nerves is soon distributed to the entire body and this delivery of impure fluids results in a stagnation in the heart, liver, kidneys and the entire excretory system. Here the mystery of rheumatism disappears. This applies to both acute and periodic or chronic rheumatism. Open the gates and let the bondman go free. I have worked accordingly and the results have been good and satisfactory.

Treatment.—In the above philosophy I have indicated the entire course for successfully treating all cases and kinds of rheumatism without regard to location. I examine every bone and every joint from the occiput to the coccyx. I think I know when an atlas is in proper articulation with the head and I know also that you know it if you have given close attention to the bony framework. By the same process we can know when all bones are in their natural places. Having this knowledge I will only say for you to carefully inhibit by gentle pressure at the back of the neck and lower part of the head. Place your fingers on the bones at the outer end of the transverse processes keeping your fingers off the muscles. By holding the ends of the fingers on the two extremities of any bone of the neck you can work with considerable force and not hurt your patient. Work gently until you find you have good articulation.

Go on with this treatment down to the coming out from the spinal cord of the brachial nerves adjusting carefully every articulation. Now we have everything in good order from the occiput to the brachial nerves and we may expect good vital living fluid to be ready for the brachial system just so soon as the cerebellum and the base of the brain have been relieved from fluids diseased by congestion, stagnation and fermentation. We must remember the vast importance of feeding the pneumogastric, the cardiac, and the sympathetic or the nutrient system of nerves with good nerve fluid which is supplied to them from the brain.

Now we are done with the bones of the neck, we will go on and remove all constricting conditions that we find in the upper dorsal. Adjust both clavicles to the normal by following the process I gave you in measles, because it is the treatment you need here and I think much repetition is useless. I know it is, if we have given the attention to anatomy that we should. Normalize every bone of the whole spine and limbs.

Of good plain nourishing food let the patient eat what he wants, and rest on such a bed as he is accustomed to and as pleases him. I look for the comfort of the patient and expect nothing from dietetics any more than I would expect a change of results by greasing the spokes of a wagon wheel. This method of treatment applies to every joint in the body affected with so-called rheumatism, and as the oldest osteopathic mechanic in the world I have here reported to you what I think is the cause of rheumatism.

CHRONIC RHEUMATISM.

Definition.—Chronic rheumatism is attended with pains in the hips, shoulders, knees, and other large joints, at times confined to one joint, at others shifting from one to another without occasioning inflammation or fever. The complaint often continues thus for a long time, and then ceases. There is no danger attendant upon it, but the patient may become lame, and is always liable to painful recurrences. Effusion of coagulable lymph is apt to occur, so as to occasion permanent thickening of the parts.

—*Dunglison*.

Symptoms.—Such painful conditions of the nerves and muscles from the first dorsal to the bottom of the foot have always been regarded as rheumatism. We know we ache and our joints hurt. Our muscles are sore. We cannot rise from a chair without producing pain and misery. Our back hurts, our heart wiggles and we are sore to some degree all over the body. We have taken the great "cure-alls" trying to get relief. The swelled condition will be in one arm, shoulder, el bow or wrist one day and in the other arm or side very soon. A similar condition of the legs occurs, first in one then the other. We have some headache, an active pulse, poor appetite, constipation or dysentery, and tenderness about the kidneys. The urine is very highly colored.

We have been faithful to the doctor's prescriptions with the hope of being relieved and after the system has been worn out the rheumatism has disappeared. The next winter it returns and we go through the same routine of misery and dope. We know the doctor's doping does us no good but much harm by getting us into the morphine habit. During the whole time the doctor never examined a bone in our body. We are sore even in hot weather. When our wagons fail to do good service we take them to the shop and the blacksmith carefully examines them, tells us what is the matter and repairs them, thus proving that he knows his business. The doctor is a mechanical failure or he would know what is wrong with the machinery of our bodies, regulate it and give us relief.

Etiology and Examination.—When a case of rheumatism comes to me for relief the first thought is, here is an effect. What has produced it? I know when the blood flows normally to and from all parts we have a healthy person without pain or misery. With this fact before my eyes, as a mechanic I begin the search for the obstructing cause. I critically examine all joints from the head to the sacrum to discover if the spine is at fault. I can find the trouble if I know my business. With this confidence and guided by the philosophy of an engineer, I examine beginning with the fifth lumbar and going downward, for in all cases of rheumatism of the lower spine and limbs, I know from long experience that we will find some variation in one or both the hips or innominates. The head of the thigh bone may be out of the socket and the capsular ligaments in a strained condition interfering with the normal flow of blood to the thigh, and I am sorry to say that it is harder work to get this fact into the head of an operator than it is to do the work and cure a half-dozen cases of sciatic and lumbar rheumatism.

I want to emphasize the importance of carefully examining the hip and adjusting it and removing the tangled condition of the muscles and ligaments around the head of the femur which causes a suppression of the blood supply and activity of the part. I care nothing for descriptive theories on rheumatism. Any man or woman suffering with this disease is better authority in a description of rheumatism than all the theoretical and laboratory experiments. In reading these theories you learn nothing because of the writer's ignorance of the mechanical laws governing healthy action of the nerve and blood supply of the lumbar region and the region of the leg and hip joint.

Treatment.—My first effort is to readjust the head of the thigh bone in the socket. With the patient sit ting erect in a chair the sound side or limb against the wall, I stand on the side of the lame leg, flex the knee and hip joint, pulling the heel towards me and pressing the knee from me to loosen all the muscles. Turning the head of the thigh bone outward, with my hand on the trochanter major I gently raise and bring the knee toward the face and placing the chin on the inside of the knee pull it toward me carrying the heel or foot across the other knee or leg. With a slight rotatory movement I let the limb come down across the sound leg at the knee making a fulcrum of the knee. With one hand on the head of the trochanter of the femur I pull gently and firmly towards the socket, holding the trochanter from me while I bring the limb to the floor from the knee. This is simple to any mechanical head, and applies to both legs.

By practicing this system of manipulation on well persons the operator can become an expert in setting hips and relieve seventy-five per cent or the cases of sciatic rheumatism of the lumbar and lower limbs. This is my procedure and is always satisfactory to the patient and myself.

In conclusion, explore and adjust all vertebrae from sacrum to occiput, also the ribs. Never spend time analyzing urine, taking temperature, applying hot and cold bags of water or telling what to eat and drink. If you remove the cause recovery will follow.

CHOREA.

Definition.—St. Vitus's dance, St. John's dance. An affection characterized by irregular and involuntary motions of one or more limbs, of the face and of the trunk. It is a disease usually occurring before puberty and is generally connected with rheumatism and often valvular disease of the heart. Its duration is long, but it is usually devoid of danger, although frequently but little under the control of medicine. The spasms do not continue during sleep. Indications of treatment are to strengthen the general system and to repress the nervous excitability.

—*Dunglison.*

Description and Etiology.—I have had experience for many years with this disturbance of motor action. The medical authors have failed to give us any authoritative information about its cause and their drug medication is an acknowledged failure. During the twenty years that I depended upon drugs I learned that the pill doctor had about settled down on the conclusion that he could use palliatives, purgatives, stimulants, blisters and so on for the spine. They all proved failures. When I concluded to take up the osteopathic telescope aided by the search—light of reason I found absolute abnormal conditions of the spinal column in various places from the occiput to the sacrum sufficient to cause these choreic movements. Since then I have treated many cases by adjusting the spinal column from end to end, and the ribs to their normal articulations, with the result that the child was relieved and the disease disappeared.

I have had patients of all ages from infancy to man hood and womanhood and the results following my treatment have been good in most cases. When the operator knows his business and does his work as he should I think that osteopathy is reliable and trustworthy in all cases and successful where there has been no surgical injury such as follows delivery by forceps, or falls or blows. I will tell you of a case which came to me early in my osteopathic work here in my own town. A young lady about sixteen years of age had suffered with chorea, according to her parent's report, since she was a little girl four or five years old. At the time she was brought to me for treatment she could not safely feed herself unless she simply used her hands in place of knife, fork or spoon. As I had met with good success in other cases by working at the spine I concluded in this case to go a little further than I had yet done and see if I could not find some abnormal condition in the spine, of some one vertebra or of the ribs. So as I sat on a chair I asked the young woman to take her place before me on her knees and between my knees with her face toward me and her arms over my shoulders. This she did with a good deal of jerking and twisting of head, spine and upper limbs. It was not long until I found several places between the fourth dorsal and the sacrum in which the vertebrae were not in their natural positions. While the patient was in this position I proceeded to adjust the entire spine as best I could with the slight experience that I had in spinal adjustment at that time. To my surprise and satisfaction complete delivery from the disease was obtained from the first treatment that I gave her and she has had no return of the chorea.

A more recent case is the one of young Paul, son of Rev. Bolton who has given the following description of it:

"My son Paul who is between seven and eight years of age was in a weak condition for six or eight months. He seemed to have poor nerve and blood supply, poor appetite, and an irritable disposition and as a climax to this condition, on July 3, 1907 he was badly scared by a dog. He ran into the house and fell full length on the floor. That evening we noticed something was wrong with him as he could not lift a glass of water to his mouth without letting it fall. The following morning his right side was so affected that he could not feed himself with that hand and he also had but very little use of his right leg. It was impossible for him to hold his head still. His speech became so much affected that it was impossible for him to make his wants known. He remained in this condition for several weeks when one morning we discovered that his left side was also affected. This left him in a very helpless condition. He was unable to walk, sit on a chair, enter into conversation with anyone or feed himself. He was always worse after his bath was given him, and usually had to be held in bed at night as he had no control over his nerves. At this stage of the disease I consulted Dr. A. T. Still who after a thorough examination pronounced the condition one of chorea and proceeded to treat him according to the Osteopathic Science. In less than six weeks my son was completely cured and is today enjoying the best of health. No other than osteopathic treatment was used."

March 25, 1908.   Signed by *Redmond A. Bolton,*
Kirksville, Mo.   Presbyterian Clergyman.

In responding to Elder Bolton's request that I call, see and give my Opinion of his little boy's condition, I found a case of the worst form of chorea, a description of which has been given by the Elder's own pen. Without any further remarks I will give you a history of my explorations for the cause which I believed existed in an abnormal condition of the spine. I found from the occiput to the sacrum variations from the normal. The fifth lumbar was far back on its articulation with the sacrum and held so by irritation and contracture of the sacro-lumbar muscles from which the nerve and blood supply was almost cut off by the position of the spine in that region. I found no abnormalities in the remaining lumbar vertebrae but at the twelfth dorsal I found a partial dislocation to the right and both ribs were down shutting off the venous drainage. Passing on up from the twelfth I found slips to the right or left until I reached the fourth. I also found the atlas drawn forward and under the occiput. I attributed the shaking or involuntary motions to the starved condition of the nervous system, the nutrient supply for the nerves, and also the cerebrospinal fluid, being shut off at the occiput. The intercostal and spinal nerves and blood-vessels were obstructed by the abnormal condition that I found in the bony framework, and from my examination and previous experience I concluded that the shortage of nerve supply resulted from abnormal conditions of the spine from the occiput on down, particularly in the region of the medulla oblongata above and as low down as the twelfth dorsal.

Treatment.—Seating myself on a chair with my patient before me on his knees, I have him throw his arms over my shoulders. I hold his body fast between my knees and adjust all variations from the truly normal between the sacrum and the occiput, being very particular with those from the sixth to the tenth dorsal. They must be absolutely correct. This treatment I give not oftener than once a week. I think it is not best to treat oftener. When properly adjusted they should be let alone thus giving Nature a chance to do her work of supplying the spinal cord with good healthy blood. By this method I have obtained good results with my patients who were twenty-five years of age or under. I have benefited older persons, straightened their spines, modified and improved the motion of their spine, arms and head. In treating the young boy of Elder Bolton who was between seven and eight years old, I began my work as I sat on a chair. The Elder brought his son to me, placed him on his knees on the floor in front of me and between my knees. As I had already made the examination to satisfy myself as to the cause of the trouble, I began my adjustment at the fifth lumbar, holding the boy tight between my knees, firmly fixing his hips, then placing my fingers on the transverse processes of the fifth I drew up and forward quite strongly with a rotatory motion to the right and left, keeping my fingers firmly on the processes until I had the fifth lumbar articulation normal. Then I came up to the region of the twelfth or floating ribs on both sides which I spread out from the spine gently and firmly in order to let the nerve and blood supply of the quadratus lumborum and the lower spinal muscles have a normal action. Then beginning at the tenth dorsal I articulated all ribs, the ninth, eighth, seventh, sixth and fifth. I saw that they were normal with their vertebrae and that the vertebrae themselves were all in line. I passed to the upper ribs and then to the clavicles both of which I found drawn back at the outer end and entirely off from their normal scapular articulations. I passed one arm under the child's arm and placed my fingers on the spinous processes next to the shoulder that I wished to adjust. While in that position I took his arm out at right angles and at this time I moved the child so as to catch the axillary part of the chest between my knees in order to hold the scapula firm while I could draw the clavicle forward to its normal articulation. Then I changed over and fixed the other scapula and clavicle after the same manner. Then I was done all but the atlas, axis and upper part of the neck which was ab normally forward, obstructing the carotid arteries on their way to supply the brain as well as the descending venous return. These I carefully adjusted in the manner already described to you. I advised the family to feed the boy when he was hungry, lay him down and let him rest when he was tired, and as he was always in a worse condition following a water bath, I advised the use of lard, almond or olive oil instead of water. I have also had other patients with this condition in its worst form who returned to normal health following the adjustment of the bony structure.

ECZEMA.

Definition.—Humid scall or tetter, moist tetter, running scall. Eruption of small vesicles on various parts of the skin, usually set close or crowded together, with more or less inflammation around their bases. The skin becomes infiltrated, the vesicles break down and exude a fluid which dries and forms crusts. There is often burning or itching and the lesions of scratching are imposed upon those peculiar to the disease. Some times there are more or less marked constitutional disturbances, though often, especially in the chronic forms, the disease is strictly local. The lesions of eczema vary greatly, and many affections of very diverse character are loosely grouped under this term. To eczema of the legs the term fluxus salinus has occasionally been given, on account of the copious secretion from it.

—Dunglison.

Etiology.—Under this heading we will include shingles or herpes zoster and facial and scalp eruptions. In dealing with skin eruptions the medical authorities give the whole list of skin affections coming under the head of eczema. (See Dunglison's classification). After we have read the medical authors and Dunglison's definition and classification we know what such and such an appearance is called and that is all that we obtain from these authorities. Outside of infections and contagions I think all of these skin disturbances are the effects of imperfect nerve and blood circulation in the superficial fascia and skin. But the producing cause of such disturbance is not given by any author. I reason that such irritating effects as we see on the skin are the result of deranged nerve and blood supply producing congestion and fermentation of the substances in the superficial fascia. There is also an inflammation of the excretory ducts of the skin. I am fully satisfied from long experience with such-eruptions as St. Anthony's fire, or facial erysipelas, that the cause is suspended nerve and blood circulation of the fascia and skin. For many years I have reasoned and practiced after the indications of this philosophy with good results as to relief and cure of skin affections. When I got the circulation (supply and drainage) normal the result was the disappearance of these effects seen in the skin.

Treatment.—I begin at the atlas and adjust it, then the neck, the dorsal, the lumbar, the sacrum and all of the ribs. My object being to open communication from the heart to the brain for nerve force and fluids and to remove every obstruction, then there can be no venous obstruction or stagnation. In order to avoid this I want the road between the brain and the heart unobstructed to abundant blood supply and venous drainage.

As the liver is often found to be congested in such patients I am very particular to adjust all vertebrae and ribs from the first to the twelfth dorsal. As we should have the excreting system do its part I adjust to perfection all lumbar articulations. Then I carefully examine the coccyx and adjust it because an abnormal coccyx may give rise to many serious diseases through pressure on the hemorrhoidal nerves, veins and arteries. I have my patient take the knee-chest position with chest on stool and adjust the spine thoroughly as described in the treatment for lumbago.

Now I lay my patient at length on the treating table, bare the back and with the heel of my hands apply friction with considerable force until I get the skin of the back from the occiput to the sacrum in a warm, red condition. I quit when I have opened the road from the brain to the coccyx so that there is no obstruction to either nerve or blood system. Such patients I treat twice a week. The expert operator soon learns to do all this work in a very short time. It is not necessary for you to worry patients by indulging in long drawn out treatments.

DROPSY.

Definition of Hydrops.—Dropsy. Abnormal collection of serous fluid in any cavity or in the areolar texture. When the areolar tissue of the whole body is more or less filled with fluid it is called anasarca or leucophlegmatia when this is local or partial it is called oedema. In encysted dropsy fluid is enclosed in a sac or cyst—dropsy of the ovarium is an instance. Dropsy may be active, consisting in an exudation of much more fluid than can normally be absorbed; or passive, arising from atony of the absorbent vessels, allowing accumulation of fluid. It may be mechanical, produced by obstruction to the circulation, as in disease of the liver. Treatment consists in using remedies which act on the various secretions, so that the demand being increased the supply will have to be increased accordingly; and in this manner the collected fluid may be taken up by the absorbents.

—Dunglison.

Etiology.—After having given you Dunglison's definition of dropsy I will say that I agree that the whole human body with all of its organs can be filled with water and if it is not passed off and out normally we have that enlarged condition in all or any part of the system known as dropsy. I think the nutrient supply of the motor nerve is not sufficient to sustain that force necessary to keep up active secretion and excretion. Also I think the nervous system of the digestive tract is not nourished sufficiently to keep up such action of the colon, peritoneum and omentum as is necessary in order that they produce or select healthy chyle from the region of the colon. Healthy chyle is the foundation-substance for the production of healthy blood. Thus I think the failure of the lower abdomen to prepare and deliver to the heart and lungs healthy chyle is one of the causes of such watery deposits as are observed and variously described under the head of dropsy.

I reason that starved nerves cannot carry on vital functioning and when the nutrient nerve system is exhausted for the want of nourishment, when the vitality of the excreting nerves is not kept up to the normal standard we have universal failure of the whole system and the deposits of water will be retained.

Examination and Treatment.—In treating patients suffering with dropsical conditions I think exploration for cause is of much more importance to the mechanic or osteopath than any amount of laboratory theories, so I will proceed to give you my method of exploration and treatment. I begin the examination of the spine at the coccyx. Then go to the sacrum, take up and explore all the lumbar, being very particular about the fourth and fifth. Then go on up exploring carefully to the eighth dorsal because I know that if the kidneys and other excretories had carried this water out of the body normally we would have had no such bulky ac cumulation as is seen and known to exist in all forms of dropsy, general or local.

I generally treat such patients on the table. I adjust all of the vertebrae cautiously, yet using considerable force with an adult patient. I am very careful to bring the eleventh and twelfth ribs into their normal places, for I want to relieve the entire renal system of nerves and blood-vessels and also the ureters from any obstructing pressure by the bony system.

Then I have my patient sit on the stool and I proceed to adjust very carefully the clavicles at both ends as I have before described. Now I carefully adjust the upper dorsal, the ribs on both sides, and the cervical vertebrae in order that there may be no pressure on the pneumogastric or any of the nerves passing from the brain or cord which are in any manner interested in the secreting or the excreting systems. I want my patient's nervous system left entirely free for good action.

I look upon it as being of the greatest importance for the lower bowel of patients in this condition, the colon in particular, to have good pure substances from which to extract chyle and other fluids necessary to be carried to the heart and the lungs and pass through the process of purifying and manufacturing normal blood which is to be distributed throughout the entire system in order that it may do its functioning of universal renovation, repair and return, maintaining the system in its original normal condition which we call health. In order to give the colon something to work on I make a gruel of flour, not starch, that is first heated to a light yellow color in order that it will not ferment. Of this I make one quart of gruel at a time and add thereto one half pint of pure cream. I inject into the colon about one half of this quantity and in a few hours' time I inject the other half. The second day following I repeat this gruel feeding or filling up the bowel with such fluid with the hope that the colon will then be able to send up to the heart pure chyle.

I have been well rewarded by this process of treatment of the bony system and the bowel as just described. In a very short time my patient's system begins to throw off the watery deposits, the swelling leaves the feet, the legs, the abdomen and the whole system. The kidneys become normal, the lungs normal, the heart normal, the brain normal, also the secretory and the excretory systems. This has been my observation and my practice and the results have been satisfactory and have taught me that much depends upon furnishing the colon with good nutritious food. Unless the case is very far advanced or the kidneys are diseased badly there is much hope for relief and for cure in such cases.

ANEMIA.

Definition.—Bloodlessness deficiency of blood opposite condition to plethora or hyperaemia. The essential character of blood in anaemia is diminution in number of the red corpuscles, also of albumin, the serum containing a disproportionate amount of water. The chief symptoms are debility, palpitation, sometimes a functional systolic murmur, and pallor of the skin and mucous membranes.

Pernicious Anaemia.—A form of extreme anaemia, advancing steadily or with slight remissions to fatal result.

—Dunglison.

Etiology.—After giving Dunglison's definitions of anemia and pernicious anemia I will say that all the writings I have read on this disease have presented to the reader the effects of observation in the chemical, the physiological and post-mortem examinations, and when all is told we find in conclusion they have simply told us what effects of the disease upon the bone, blood, nerve and other tissues they have observed. From these effects they all agree that the disease is the result of confused functioning of the whole organic system, if I rightly comprehend their conclusion.

So far as I know, no previous author has ever claimed that as a result of falls, injuries or other causes the bony framework is in an abnormal condition and that this in itself could operate to produce and. bring about this condition known as pernicious anemia. No medical author claims to have discovered a specific for the cure of this disease, but all acknowledge that the cause is not known.

Now I will ask the mechanic what sort of medicine should be administered when all authors have agreed the cause of the disease is unknown? Should the osteopath set aside his mechanical knowledge which is based upon the anatomical and physical truth that obstruction to both blood and nerve action exists prior to such manifestation and that his remedy in this disease and his success in treatment depends wholly upon his ability to adjust and to leave the body in such a condition that the normal nerve and blood supply has no obstruction by variation of either bone, ligament or muscle? My conclusion is that all of the benefit which I have given such patients has followed as a result of normal action brought about by adjusting the body to such a condition that the natural processes of blood production, of repair and so on were obtained.

Examination and Treatment.—Such cases of pernicious anemia as have come to me for osteopathic treatment have generally suffered previously from some other disease such as an infectious fever, and have gone through a course of medical treatment and were far advanced in this disease before they applied to me for relief. I always begin my exploration of the entire spinal column of these patients at the sacrum. I adjust its articulations with both innominates, with the coccyx and with the fifth lumbar. I search carefully about the hip joints to see that there is no impingement of nerves or vessels produced by contracted muscles. I carefully adjust the gluteal system and all of the joint ligaments until they are normally free, and I never leave this section until I know it is right. I want no "may-be-so's," "possibly's," or "however's," but I want mechanical knowledge used and applied to correct the structures. I want the downward current of the spinal cord to be absolutely undisturbed from its origin to the termination of the cauda equina, the sacral nerves and all other nerves of vital interest in and about the sacrum.

Now we will proceed upward from the articulation of the sacrum and the fifth lumbar, examining the entire lumbar region carefully, adjusting any and all variations in this division of the spine. We should be careful to adjust the eleventh and twelfth ribs on both sides of the spine because they are often held down and back by the quadratus lumborum muscles and the ligaments beneath them and are irritating the whole renal system. We want and must have good work done by the kidneys and we know it cannot be done when the ribs are in the condition described.

Having adjusted the eleventh and twelfth ribs we will proceed upwards adjusting every vertebra and rib until we get to the upper dorsal. Here we should carefully examine with mechanical skill in order that we may know that the fifth, sixth, seventh and eighth ribs and the dorsal vertebrae are absolutely in their normal position, having no "may-be-so's," "possibly so," or "however," about it. This is no place for foolishness because in this region the great splanchnic nerves branch off and pass to the solar plexus. We want the semilunar ganglia to do their work without hindrance. We want to get the patient out of this condition and we should put in our best effort on this region faith fully. We have but little time to spend analyzing urine, blood, lymph—or any other fluid substance of the body because we think life is too precious to dillydally in laboratory work when the structures are out of order, or before we have made all adjustments from the ah normal. We should find the producing cause and proceed to remove it.

Having finished our work with the fourth ribs and the dorsal vertebrae, we should go on up higher and bring every bone into its proper place and in line—the upper ribs, both collar bones and the shoulder blades. I say collar bone and shoulder blades because I am talking to mechanics and I aim to use the language of a mechanic. Now adjust every point of abnormality found to exist in the cervical vertebrae up to and including the articulation with the occiput. Examine the hyoid bone. See that it is normal, not too high nor too low. Then the inferior maxilla and make sure that it articulates properly on both sides, and that the blood in the vessels just back of its angle has free and uninterrupted circulation. Open up the ureters by the method already given you—with the flat of your hands laid on the abdomen just above the symphysis and then slowly drawn up towards the kidneys.

ADDISON'S DISEASE.

Definition.—Bronzed-skin disease; suprarenal cachexia; the leading characteristics are anaemia, general languor and debility, remarkable feebleness of the heart's action, irritability of the stomach, and a peculiar bronzed skin, first described by Dr. Thomas Addison, of London, as connected with a diseased condition of the suprarenal capsules; death occurs from exhaustion.

—Dunglison.

Etiology.—After the osteopath has read the medical writers' definitions and treatment he has gotten about all the information that they have been able to report. Dunglison has given a list of symptoms the cause of which the medical writers say is unknown. Autopsies show effects only because the work of destruction was complete before the knife and microscope were consulted. Invariably medical authors tell us in substance that there is no hope for recovery, but death must be expected, as a general thing, in two or three years.

In all medical literature that I have perused I find only one point that is of any benefit to the osteopathic mechanic and that point is found in the medical statistics which report that about ninety per cent of those who have been affected with Addison's disease are laborers. If this be true and post-mortems show the semilunar ganglia, the suprarenal capsule, the kidney and many other organs of the abdomen to be in an abnormal condition, then, as mechanics, we are led to reason that the cause of the organic effects just stated must precede such conditions. And in order to make a successful hunt for the cause, and knowing that at least ninety per cent of the sufferers are of the laboring class, without any further argument I will direct the student to the spinal column to seek there and find in the abnormal conditions existing and due to strains in the articulations of the spine and ribs, a sufficient cause for all the trouble.

Examination.—In all such cases I have always found on examination some variation from the truly normal in both spine and ribs, particularly-in the region from the first dorsal down to the twelfth dorsal and even as low as the fifth lumbar. Accompanying such diseases I find as a general thing the ribs out of their proper articulation with the transverse processes. They are generally below and often pushed back and between the two processes.

By the results I have gotten in anemia, dropsy, constipation, kidney trouble, and so on, after making the adjustments as outlined, I have proven to my satisfaction that if I wanted to find the cause of this organic disturbance I must seek for it in the abnormal condition of the spine and ribs, particularly in the upper dorsal and axillary regions. Here we will find much variation, the ribs being above or below their processes, with much curvature of spine and neck, generally to the right. Then we get contracture which I think is a cause producing disturbances and enlargement; at least, I have found such to be the condition in all cases. In my observation of diseased conditions of the lung, pleurae, heart, liver, spleen, stomach, bowels, kidneys, uterus, etc., I expect to find bony variations of the framework.

When I searched I found the cause and invariably gave relief if I used the judgment and skill of a mechanic; if not, I got no good results. With this short report I will give you what I consider the only remedy for Addison's disease, that can be given with any hope of either palliation or cure.

Treatment.—As I have already given careful instructions how to adjust all the bones of the spine, I will not repeat any further than to say to the operator, you must begin with the atlas and carefully adjust its articulation with the head. We want blood to go to the brain, do its work and come back. We must have a clean sweep for the artery and also for the venous system to and from the head.

Now we have articulated the atlas with the occiput we will pass on down. Articulate the atlas with the axis. Go on and articulate every cervical vertebra with its fellows both above and below it. Then articulate the seventh cervical with the first dorsal. Now adjust both clavicles. Be careful in your adjustment of the upper four ribs. They must articulate properly with their processes. Sometimes they fall off or are pushed above their processes. Pull them back into place. Pull the clavicles into their proper articulation at both the sternal and the scapular ends. Manipulate the arm and scapula as we must have normal axillary supply and drainage and we must leave it all in good order. Now go on down the spine and look for lateral variations. We will very likely find convex lateral bulging on one side with concavity of the opposite side. Correct these vertebrae and ribs that are at fault. Go on down to the eleventh and twelfth dorsal. Right here we are likely to find the floating ribs thrown off and lying nearly parallel with the spine just back of the kidneys. The quadratus lumborum muscles are attached to the twelfth ribs and the ilia. With the fingers behind them pull them down and forward, adjust them and loosen up the ribs.

Now we will go on to the lumbar vertebrae. Take out all the twists, convexities, and other variations from a normal lumbar spine. Adjust the fifth lumbar in its articulation with the sacrum. As I told you before, we should raise the lower bowel carefully up out of the pelvis and free all the structures here that by being cramped could in any way cause interference in the normal circulation of the abdominal nerve and blood supply. Have your patient take the knee-chest position on the floor, breast on the stool. Come up behind him with your knees spread out. Take your patient's hips between your knees, then begin at the fifth lumbar and place your thumbs on the transverse processes and hold them firmly. Now move your knees with a twisting motion, articulate each vertebra of the whole lumbar—the fourth, the third, the second and the first. Give this treatment in these cases about two or four days apart according to the patient's condition. Another method: I have patient get on his knees before me with his hips between my knees, his arms around my neck, and I proceed to adjust the whole spine while in that position. Many other positions are good. Our object should be a well corrected spine. Let your patient eat good plain wholesome food and plenty of it, and take such exercise as is agreeable.

In conclusion I will say that many of my patients report that they have never been physically strong since they were vaccinated with impure vaccine matter. Thus we have the effects to combat, and our only hope is to adjust and keep the bony framework all in line so that all impurities will have a chance to pass off and out.

DIABETES.

Definition.—Disease characterized by great augmentation, and often manifest alteration, in the secretion of urine, with excessive thirst and progressive emaciation. wo species are usually described—diabetes in sipidus and diabetes mellitus the former being simply a superabundant discharge of limpid urine not containing sugar; the latter—saccharine diabetes—falls under the definition given above. The quantity of urine dis charged in the twenty-four hours is sometimes excessive, amounting to 30 pints and upward, each pint containing sometimes 2¼ oz. of saccharine matter. The exciting causes are often found in diseases of the nervous centers, tumors, and injuries, especially those involving the fourth ventricle.

—Dunglison.

Etiology.—I will not wear out the patience of the osteopath by rehearsing what medical authors have said further than to state that they report they know nothing of the cause or cure of diabetes. On examination I have found variations from the normal generally beginning with the ninth dorsal. Then I carefully examine and adjust every section of spine to the sacrum and coccyx, also the eleventh and twelfth ribs on both sides. These variations act powerfully on the excretory system and excite and irritate the solar plexus which gives off branches to the abdominal excretory system. This condition of the solar plexus is but an effect for which there is a cause. There is something wrong with the great splanchnic either at is origin at about the fifth rib or in its course, extending and passing through the diaphragm and on to the solar plexus. I think the semilunar ganglia fail to do their part in nourishing the solar plexus.

I generally find the first dorsal vertebra extremely far back on the second producing a twisted condition of the base of the second on the facets of the third. As a result there is lateral curvature of the spine. The curvature excites an irritation between the fifth and sixth intercostal nerves extending to the semilunar ganglia by way of the great splanchnic which continues the irritation to the solar plexus. Irritated branches from the solar plexus reach the renal system producing heat and great thirst for water, which generally subside when the spine from the first to the eighth dorsal is properly adjusted and normal action takes the place of confusion.

Examination and Treatment.—We want light on this subject. It matters not what we call the condition, but we want to know its cause. We should explore to find the variations of coccyx, sacrum, lumbar and dorsal vertebrae, ribs, hip joints and both innominates. I find a coccyx off, a sacrum pushed out and backwards at the articulation with the lumbar, putting both in nominates on a strain. Partial dislocations of the head of the femur occur producing strains, irritation, and soreness of the lumbar region. Scrutinize the condition of the hip joints. In other chapters I have told you how to adjust the spine and lower limbs.

Give your patient plenty of good food. If he wants sugar or breakfast bacon, allow him to eat them. The bacon oils the digestive tract, and I have for many years reasoned that the patient should be fed sweet substances and honey in particular. The sugar being found in the urine is to me an evidence that it has not been appropriated to the use of the system as it should, so give your patient honey in abundance, all that the system will tolerate. Keep skimmed milk away from your patient, but fresh, rich buttermilk may be given. Be sure to gently draw the stomach and bowels from the right side to the left taking off all pressure from the solar plexus. I have given relief to all my patients and entirely cured many. This applies to patients before the collapse occurs. When a patient comes to me in a collapsed condition, I do the best I can, hoping to give some relief and lengthen their days.

SCURVY.

Definition.—A disease resembling purpura, and due mainly to the use of improper food. It is marked by large ecchymoses or petechiae, which may ulcerate, swollen and ulcered gums, and an irregular fever, with great weakness. It oftenest affects mariners and those who use salted meats and few or no vegetables.

—Dorland.

Etiology.—As far as history goes as it is given by the best authors, scurvy is an effect following a monotonous and a bad diet of cured meats or of impure food stuff, and the disease generally entirely disappears when fresh vegetables, fresh meats, fruits and other acid substances become a part of the diet.

Personally I have had very little opportunity to make an acquaintance with scurvy. According to the best authors there has been very little opportunity in the United States for doctors of any school to make its acquaintance, but all agree that such foods as armies are sometimes forced to use for the soldiers have been to a large degree lacking in fresh fruits and vegetables as well as fresh meats, and the meager diet has brought about such a condition that lime preponderates in the system and produces the poisonous condition which it requires the acids of fruits and vegetables to counteract. I consider it the effect of a poison requiring an antidote. The poisonous cause being alkali and the necessary counteracting antidote being fruit, sour milk and vegetable acids.

Treatment.—In addition to the radical change in diet I would give my scurvy patients thorough osteopathic spinal treatments, beginning at the lumbar vertebrae and making a careful and thorough examination of each vertebra, adjusting to the normal every one found at any variance with its neighbor either above or below. I would extend this work up to and including the atlas, making sure that there is perfect freedom for both nerves and blood-vessels to and from the brain. I carry out this method of treatment every few days, my object being to get rid of the over-plus of lime from the system and prepare the entire excretory apparatus to do good work in passing it off and out.

DRUNKENNESS.

Definition.—Acute alcoholic intoxication.

—Dunglison.

Is it a disgrace for a man to drink alcohol, brandy or whisky when he has a great thirst for such drinks? Would it not be cruel to turn such a patient away as though he were a criminal and you would be disgraced to be seen in his company? Is he diseased? Does his thirst for drink tell us to search for the cause? Notwithstanding it was the ruination of his home and all the joy of his loved ones, let us say that alcohol has been the drunkard's friend relieving him in his affliction. Was that whisky his friend? I say yes, but the doctor failed to see in that man's thirst the finger of Nature pointing to the cause of this cry for whisky. This thirst is because of the failure of the system to furnish its own healthy fluids which, when shut off by any cause leave a demand for a substitute. In these patients this demand is satisfied by alcoholic stimulants, so we have a sick man to consider instead of a drunk man.

Is it not reasonable to conclude that the alcohol drinker is a sick man, one whose acts should tell us that he has had by accident, strain or otherwise, a suspension of nerve and blood supply to the pancreas and spleen, and that the taste for alcohol will disappear with the return of the normal nerve and blood supply to these organs? I think whisky is the drunkard's friend because it gives him temporary relief from the oppressive action of the lime and chalk that are retained in his system, producing an abnormal thirst. If the doctor reasons from effect to cause it will be his friend in diagnosis, and he will find a temporary paralysis of the nerves of the spleen, pancreas and liver, the pancreatic juice not being sufficient in quantity to supply the system with the necessary acids to keep the body free from chalk and lime. Drunkenness is no disgrace but is proof that the man has a disease, and the failure in the free circulation of his blood has allowed his liver and spleen to retain chalk, lime and earthy substances, and has prevented the manufacturing of healthy fluids whose work is to keep the chalk and lime in a fluid condition and pass them off through the excretory system. The normal nerve and blood supply has been deranged by the variations from the normal articulation of spine and ribs, particularly in the region of the fifth, sixth, seventh and eighth ribs on the left Side (often on the right side also).

Treatment.—About twenty-five years ago I came to the conclusion that the desire for alcohol was an effect, the cause of which was surely somewhere in the spinal cord. At about that time a friend asked me to go with him into a saloon and have a drink of whisky. He was a blacksmith who drank regularly three times a day. I told him no, and began to examine his ribs and spine from the lower lumbar to the occiput. I found the ribs in the region of his left shoulder pushed upward. I threw his arm up putting the ribs on a strain and placed them back into position, and then said to him, "Now go into the saloon and come back, and if you do not turn sick at the smell of liquor I will pay for the whisky." He went into the saloon and came back to me in a few minutes saying that he had to come out of the saloon because he turned very sick. I met him often afterwards for seven years and he told me that he never drank a drop after that one treatment.

I was so much encouraged at the result obtained with him that I treated several others and got sober men for my work. I reasoned that the condition of their spines and ribs brought on the disease, a thirst for whisky. The osteopath should always treat such men with kindness and adjust all of the ribs on the left side in order to reach the pancreas, spleen, solar plexus and other nerves that become disabled previous to the appearance of that thirst. I will leave the subject here and hope that the osteopath will go on and on and set the bondman free from that effect, thirst for alcohol.

SUNSTROKE.

Definition.—Insolation, or thermic fever; a condition produced by exposure to the sun, and marked by convulsions, coma, and a very high temperature of the skin.

—*Dorland*.

Etiology.—I think an over—accumulation of venous blood in the brain produces the effect known as sun stroke. The heat overcomes the normal action of the vessels to and from the brain and venous congestion is the result.

Treatment.—With the patient upon the back I place a broad board lengthwise under the body. Elevate the head of the board at least one foot to facilitate the return of blood by its own weight. Draw head and neck well up. Keep the jugular system well open from head to heart. Place a towel wrung out of cold water upon the head, another over the heart. Place a sheet wrung out of cold water upon the back of the patient to establish venous drainage and contracture. Beginning at the ninth dorsal open up the entire spinal system with a view of having the kidneys act normally. Never apply ice in these cases because the shock is too great. Sixty degrees Fahrenheit is cold enough temperature. Raise bowels and all viscera out of the pelvis with the patient on his side, in order to establish arterial and venous drainage of the renal system. Give patient plenty of fresh air, and cold water to drink. Keep stimulants away and depend upon quieting down the venous and nervous systems. By this procedure the osteopath will have satisfactory results if called in time.

HYPERMOBILITY OF THE SPINE.

Hypermobility, or the condition in which the joints of the spine and lower limbs become loose, is an effect following the stoppage of nutrition to the nerves of motion. The joints move too freely and in persons so affected there is a swinging, uncontrollable condition of the spine and limbs. The spine below the fourth dorsal is the part chiefly affected.

Examination and Treatment.—On examination I have found serious lateral deviations, the facets of the different vertebrae being far to the right or left. There has been some fall or injury that has pushed the upper facet far enough to the right or left to produce a lock of the vertebrae and inhibit the supply of nutrition to the spinal cord at this point.

My object is to explore very carefully from the first to the eighth dorsal and ascertain exactly where the lock is. I place my patient's breast at the end of the table with a pillow between breast and table and al low the head and upper part of the chest to hang over the end of the table. With the hand on the neck I bend the head downward gently and from right to left which pulls the facets apart, and with my other hand on the spinous processes it is an easy matter to adjust the articulations. After this I let the patient rest a few days, then adjust all articulations below, including the sacrum and hips.

By this method I expect to get normal action of the spine and limbs. This will follow the return of nutrition to its normal condition which depends upon an unobstructed nerve and blood supply to the spine from the occiput to the sacrum. For thirty years this has been my procedure with the result that the spine returned to its normal condition.

CONTAGIOUS DISEASES
AND FEVERS

CONTAGION.

Definition of Contact.—State of two bodies touching each other. In the theory of contagious diseases we distinguish immediate or direct contact, as when we touch a patient laboring under such disease; mediate or indirect contact, when we touch objects that have touched him.

—Dunglison.

Definition of Contagion.—Transmission of a disease from one person to another by direct or indirect contact. Also at one time applied to the supposed action of miasmata arising from dead animal or vegetable matter, bogs, fens, etc. Contagion and infection are generally esteemed synonymous. Frequently, however, the latter is applied to disease not produced by contact, as measles, etc., while contagion is used for those that require positive contact, as itch, syphilis, etc. Diseases which are produced only by contagion are said to have their origin in specific contagion or infection, as smallpox, cowpox, syphilis, etc.

—Dunglison.

It is not necessary for the osteopath to enter into the discussion of the unanswerable question of how a contagious disease gets possession of the person. A knowledge of this process has long since been pronounced by the medical world an impossibility. Seekers have labored to ascertain and know just how a contagion gets possession of or is communicated from one person to another and all agree that they have totally failed to obtain this knowledge. Thirty-four years ago I dropped all hope of ever being able to tell the how and why of the contagious properties of smallpox, chickenpox, mumps, measles and whooping-cough, and how they proceed to get possession of the body of a healthy person and begin their torture and go on to recovery or death. Hence I began at that time to search as an anatomical mechanic to find out just what it is that interferes with the venous, arterial and lymphatic vessels and the place or point where a stoppage of the normal flow of their fluids is produced. What is the cause of the greater arterial excitement? Why in all such diseases do the deep and superficial glandular systems of the neck, spine and fascia become filled up, and why do these glandular systems not unload or carry off these fluids in place of retaining them until stag nation, fermentation, inflammation and death do their work?

The engineer has to control the engine that produces smallpox, chickenpox, measles, mumps, whooping cough, diphtheria, laryngitis, pharyngitis, tonsillitis, tumors of the nose, diseases of the tongue, throat, mouth, eyes and all the organs of the face and head. As the discoverer of osteopathy I will say that in my practice and from my observation I have noticed that the portion of the nervous system most affected, is situated in the region between the diaphragm and the foramen magnum.

The osteopath should prepare himself and be governed accordingly if he wishes to be a critic in explorations for the cause or causes of such diseases as are named above, with the addition of those of the heart, pleurae and lungs. While these diseases are different in effects, appearances and names, yet they attack and execute their work by overcoming the harmony of nerve and blood action between the base of the skull and the diaphragm. With this introduction I shall proceed to deal with such diseases and give the reader the benefit of such discoveries as I have made as to cause, relief or cure.

GERMS AND PARASITES.

Definition of Germ.—Rudiment of new being, not yet developed or still adherent to the mother. Spore or living particle which has been detached from already existing living matter. A microorganism.

Definition of Parasite.—(Parasiteo, to eat in the house of). Organism, animal or vegetable, living during the whole or part of its existence in or on the body of some other organism, the latter being called the host.

Human parasites are both animal and vegetable. The former include Entozoa (animals living in the interior of the human body) and Ectozoa (those which infest the exterior). Vegetable parasites are the Entophyta and Epiphyta, the former existing in the interior of the body, the latter on the exterior. The simplest arrangement of entozoa includes Coelelmintha (koilos, hollow, helmins, worm), hollow worms; Stereimintha (stereos, solid), solid worms; and accidental parasites.

—Dunglison.

We can analyze the blood or sputum and guess at what the patient ate three months ago. We find germs which are fat, lean, round, long, short and all shapes. I think we spend too much time in that kind of work. We have no controversy with scientists over the fact that germs are found in the system. This was proven many years ago. The germs must have suitable conditions or they fail to appear in dangerous numbers. First, they must have dead flesh to eat or they will die. It has been proven that germs of different kinds have been found in diseased lungs, diseased kidneys, and in other diseased organs and parts of the system. They appear in great numbers in parts of the system that have given way after a long continuation of fevers or in prostration that accompanies the disease in which they are found. A few germs have been reported to have been found in healthy persons. We are well satisfied that there was some failure of the blood, Nature's reliable germicide, to reach and repair and hold healthy possession of that part of the body in which the germ has been found. We will stick to the belief that Nature's chemistry can produce and apply the substance that will destroy any germ that appears in the various kinds of disease in which it is claimed they are found. Not only can

Nature's chemistry destroy the germs but it can disorganize and pass away unnatural accumulations of lime. In diseases of the liver, kidney, thyroid gland and many other organs, lime accumulates only when the activities of sensation, motion and nutrition are suspended by some obstruction between the heart and nervous system and the accumulated local excrescence. Thus we have unbounded faith that Nature's chemistry is the doctor and the only one on whom we can depend for relief. Nature abounds with remedies necessary for her use in all conditions.

We will try to assist the reader to fully comprehend what we mean by germs. I believe they are universally the products of decomposition. When a tree dies in a forest it ceases to produce leaves, flowers and fruit. It begins to live a new life which is just as active as the life it lived when producing the tree. The second life or condition is ordinarily known as de composition. It goes on and on until complete disintegration of all atoms is accomplished. After the tree has been as we say dead twelve months we see that it is not dead but actively producing another form of being commonly known as frogstool. Under the microscope we see a perfect system in the preparation of Nature to produce this spongy growth. We see finely formed fibers and we see a difference in the different parts of this spongy growth. Some of it is as coarse as the fibers of red muscle in the animal, some has the appearance of liver, kidney, lung, secretion, excretion, arterial, venous and all of the systems in the animal life except locomotion. The philosopher will see at once that he has before him the system of a living, acting object, whose business it is to collect material and conduct a chemical manufacturing process which prepares the elements and conducts them to their proper position and adjusts them under the most exacting laws of construction.

But I want to draw the attention of the observer of this process to the fact that the dead condition of the tree or log had to be complete before the process of the new life could go on and on and start the work of forming those tumors. This I think should be very valuable to the osteopath who is taught to dread the germs which I think he should dread until he learns how to proceed and keep the tree in a healthy condition and keep it out of all chances of local and general death. If you wound a tree in the forest it goes on through all of the steps from the wound to gangrene and death. The osteopath must overcome similar wounds in the body by adjusting the parts in the locality of an organ injured. He is warned to keep the blood or sap in a condition to be delivered and appropriated. He must do this by first attaining a correct knowledge of form, force, supply and function and then by skill he can maintain a normal condition of the human body. Then he will have no tumors or unnatural deposits to be turned over to the surgeon's knife.

MEASLES.

Definition.—A contagious eruptive fever with coryza and catarrhal symptoms. The period of incubation is about two weeks, and the disease begins with fever, chills, conjunctivitis, severe coryza, and frequently bronchitis, causing cough and frontal headache. The eruption appears on the fourth day on the forehead, cheeks, and back of the neck, spreading thence over the body. It consists of small dark-pink macules in crescentic groups, which frequently become confluent. After two or three days the eruption begins to fade, and is followed in one or two weeks by desquamation. The symptoms increase with the eruption and decrease with the disappearance of it, convalescence beginning in the second week. The disease is extremely contagious and affects chiefly the young, one attack usually conferring immunity. Measles is prone to lead to complications, the chief of which are pneumonia, bronchitis, phthisis, and otitis media.

—Dorland.

Symptoms.—This disease is very much like smallpox and chickenpox in its effect on the human system. We have such symptoms as headache, backache, fever and skin eruption. The kidneys cease to throw off. The skin ceases to discharge its excretions. The lungs thicken. The voice changes. The neck, face and eyes are congested. The eruption generally appears on head, face, limbs and body in succession until the entire body is covered and then lasts but a few days. The eruption is so well known by all persons that I do not think it necessary to take up your time with any of the theories which in and of themselves are useless.

Etiology.—Measles is a condition or effect produced by a poisonous, infectious and contagious gas, so far as we know. The question is not what is the cause, but what part of the body does this poisonous substance affect? It irritates the whole constrictor system of the human body and closes the excretory gates so tight that the foul gases cannot pass out from the body through the porous system. All infectious dis eases such as measles, mumps, smallpox, chickenpox and other rashes are simply an exhibit of the method that Nature uses to get rid of deadly poisons that should have passed through the excretory pipes or ducts. We conclude that when the fluids of the body are stopped in the fascia, organs and other parts of the system, stagnation, fermentation, heat and general confusion will follow until the system grows hot enough to produce a finer gas or cold enough to relax the skin and let those poisonous fluids pass out and off.

The osteopath sees at once that this irritating poison is the cause that produces inflammatory action which converts the fluids of the fascia into pus. The local gangrenous spots of the skin, when suppurated, make openings for the pus to leave the superficial fascia and pass out of the system. Nature has many methods of renovating the body from the deadly poisons resulting from stagnation, decomposition, etc., and this is one of them.

The medical doctor reasons that he has a chemical poison to contend with and hunts for a chemical antidote to antagonize the poison. He experiments with both internal and external applications. The mechanic stands by and beholds the unsuccessful combat and by the death of the patient he is convinced that medication is an absolute failure. Some patients with great vitality survive but dependence upon the administration of medicine by the most learned experimenters is not trustworthy.

The mechanic asks, "What is the irritating cause that produces such universal interference with the excretory system and allows the deadly decomposition to get in its work?" The mechanical philosopher must reason from effect to cause. Then he will raise the lever that holds the fluids in stagnation. When he does this he is like an engineer who opens the mud valve and lets all impurities pass from the boilers. In comparison he says, "This human engine must have the mud valve raised and give the boilers a chance to produce pure and healthy, steam or all will be wrecked."

Examination.—We will begin our exploration for the cause of the thickening of the muscles and tissues of the neck at the base of the brain, and continue to the sternum and the intercostal ligaments and muscles covering the upper four ribs around to their union with the spine. I always find soreness and much contracture in this locality, stopping the fluids until inflammatory action gets in its work. Thus the importance of having the blood pass without obstruction from the heart, up the neck, into and out of the head and face. No inhibition by irritation, contraction or congestion should be allowed to hinder the perfect flow of blood. During all examinations of such patients I have found muscular contractions at the union of the neck with the head. I reason that the arterial blood is delivered to and retained in the face and head and all its organs. There is no difficulty so far, in blood or nerve action, but here are a congested face, eyes and head. The question is why are they presenting this congested condition? I reason that the blood that was driven into the cranium by arterial force is retained there because the venous system is unable to return the blood from this region back to the heart. Then why has the venous system failed? Your answer is, there is muscular contracture or pressure upon the venous system.

Thus we know that outside of the chemical action that the virus produces, pressure on the vessels that should drain the head and face is the cause of the in ability of the venous system to carry its blood back to the heart. I have given you my reason and experience and told you the things that I have observed for many years in my care of patients suffering with measles whom I have uniformly relieved by osteopathic treatment.

Treatment.—I carefully adjust the upper part of the neck, the atlas, axis and all points in the cervical and on down as low as the fourth dorsal. Then the ribs and collar bones. I lay my patient on his back or side, place my left hand at the occiput, my right on the forehead and carefully adjust the atlas and the axis and all the bones of the neck from any abnormal condition that may be found to exist. I also bring the clavicles forward at both ends in order to take off all pressure from the muscles, nerves and blood-vessels of the neck. I do this by spreading the arms apart while my patient is lying on his back, using a book or surgical pillow um der the scapulae to hold them in a stationary condition. I bring the outer end of the clavicle forward on the acromian process using considerable strength. Then I bring the upper ribs forward to their normal place.

Now I stand at the head of my patient and inhibit the occipital nerves after which I lay my hand flat alongside of the neck over the congested glands and muscles and follow down to the seventh cervical vertebra. Because of the constriction behind the jaw it is important to bring the inferior maxilla forward and the atlas and axis backward. In measles and all such diseases the same condition of contracture exists in the axilla. The arms must be raised and the axillary regions freed at once and kept so. While the patient is lying on the bed I generally sit down on the side of it and take the arm between the wrist and the elbow, straighten it out at right angles with the body and with my other hand under the scapula on the same side I catch on to the ribs gently but with fairly good force draw them upward towards the sternum. I do this in order that the pressure of the ribs can be taken off the inferior cervical ganglion also to let the axillary circulation have perfect freedom which I think is of great importance in measles.

Now go down to the kidneys and stop at the eleventh and twelfth ribs and pull them forward and up using gentle force in order to take all pressure off the renal nerves, veins and arteries. From there go to the region of the bladder and bring both hands together just above the symphysis making a gentle but firm pressure for a short time. Then move your hands up towards the kidneys. Do this in order to overcome any constriction that would interfere with the delivery of the urine from the kidneys through the ureters and down into the bladder. Turn the patient on the right side and gently draw the stomach and bowels toward the left in order to give freedom to the solar plexus, the aorta and all nerves from the solar plexus supplying the organs of the abdomen. The aorta furnishes the blood, the solar plexus the nerves, the venous and excretory systems carry away the impurities through the excretory ducts. Do this work as a mechanic of thought and skill and the results will be good and satisfactory to both the doctor and his patient.

For a few days keep the patient in a room reason ably dark and give the ordinary diet of plain, nutritious, easily digested foods. In my experience I have generally left this question with the mother. This has been my method of procedure for many years in the treatment of patients suffering with measles and without the loss of a single patient. This same result is the report of the graduates of my school. In small pox, chickenpox, measles, diphtheria and scarlet fever there is a great similarity of the conditions produced throughout the glandular system.

WHOOPING-COUGH.

Definition.—Pertussis; an infectious disease characterized by catarrh of the respiratory tract and peculiar paroxysms of cough ending in a prolonged crowing or whooping respiration. After an incubation-period of about two weeks the catarrhal stage begins with slight fever, sneezing, running at the nose and a dry cough. In a week or two the paroxysmal stage begins with the characteristic paroxysmal cough. This consists of a deep inspiration followed by a series of quick short coughs, continuing until the air is expelled from the lungs. During the paroxysm the face becomes cyanosed, the eyes injected, and the veins distended. The cough frequently induces vomiting and in severe cases, epistaxis or other hemorrhage. The close of the paroxysm is marked by a long-drawn, shrill, whooping inspiration, due to spasmodic closure of the glottis. The number of paroxysms varies from ten or twelve to forty or fifty in twenty-four hours. This stage lasts from three to four weeks, and is followed by the stage of decline during which the paroxysms grow less frequent and less violent, and finally cease. The disease is most frequently met with in children, is much more prevalent in cold weather, and is very contagious, the virus being apparently associated with the sputum. The disease is apt to be complicated with catarrhal pneumonia, pulmonary collapse, emphysema, convulsions, and hemorrhages into the eye, ear, or brain, and severe cases are sometimes followed by chronic bronchitis, tuberculosis, or nephritis.

—Dorland.

Etiology.—I will leave the how and why of the contagious nature of whooping-cough just where the medical world has left them, an unsolved mystery. But for the benefit of the osteopath who wishes to relieve the suffering, I will make an effort to tell something of the effect which is produced and the results secured under osteopathic treatment.

Prognosis.—The medical prognosis is almost without hope of relief in whooping-cough, especially with complications. In my practice I have been well acquainted with whooping-cough and treated it for many years according to medical methods and came to the same conclusion that other medical doctors did. They said "Whooping-cough is whooping-cough and is a self-limiting disease," then turned the patient over to the mother and she was told to do the best she could.

In 1874 when I began to reason upon the mechanical construction of the human body I proceeded to hunt for the cause or causes that produced such phenomena. I soon found heavy spasmodic contractions of the muscles of the sides of the neck as well as of all the thoracic muscles as low down as the fifth, sixth and sometimes the seventh rib. I found these muscles very sensitive, sore and rigid, drawing the clavicles and sternum back on to the respiratory nerves, hence the mechanical cause of the irritation was very plain to me and relief as well as shortening of the period of the attack was certain to follow the adjustment of the structures. If you get the case early you can generally stop its course at once. As a rule we can terminate the course of whooping-cough in from three to fifteen days.

Examination.—In making my examination of a patient suffering with whooping-cough I begin with the front of the thorax. The sternum, the upper ribs, the clavicles, the upper dorsal and all of the cervical vertebrae are to be carefully examined. Also all of the musculature of the neck and thorax are to be thoroughly looked after and all contractions reduced and relaxed and the head is to be adjusted on the atlas and all the vessels and nerves set free.

Treatment.—In my work with the little sufferers I proceed to adjust all of the bones of the upper chest, the clavicles, the sternum, the spine and particularly the atlas. I am careful to see that the atlas is in its articulation with the occiput in order to secure a free passage for the blood to and from an irritated brain. I also inhibit at two points just inside and back of the transverse processes of the atlas. I do this by using gentle firm pressure with the flat of my fingers at those points, the patient sitting in front of me. Relaxation of the muscles of the neck follows, respiration is soon reduced and the child gets down and goes on with its play. At first I was surprised to find that many children would be entirely relieved in from three to fifteen days. When you think of whooping-cough, think as a mechanic thinks concerning the machine over which he has charge. Do your work accordingly and often you will be surprised at your results which will be far beyond your expectations.

DIPHTHERIA.

Definition.—(Diphtheria, skin or membrane). Diphtheritis, an infectious disease characterized by profound vital depression and the formation, through exudation and necrosis, of a false membrane, usually on the tonsils and pharynx, but affecting sometimes the mouth, nose, or larynx. The membrane formed is grayish white and adherent, leaving, when detached, a raw surface. Ulceration and gangrene sometimes follow, and other organs, as the glands, become involved. The symptoms, of course, vary with the part affected, whether the seat of it be the fauces, larynx, or nose. In about one-sixth of the cases diphtheritic paralysis occurs, usually in the pharynx. The disease is due to the presence of a specific microorganism, the Klebs-Loeffler bacillus, and the constitutional symptoms are caused by the action of the toxins elaborated by this microbe.

—Dunglison.

Etiology.—After we have read what the most eminent physicians have to say as to the cause or causes that produce the deadly malady known as diphtheria we are left, as I understand it, without a compass to direct us to any philosophical conclusion as to its cause or cure.

We know that diphtheria is more prevalent in the fall, winter and spring than in the summer season. We know that it appears more frequently in cold, wet, chilly weather; and more often when the wind is from the east than from any other point. We know that after such continuous damp cold spells that the patient is attacked and presents some or all of the symptoms that have been enumerated, or that can be found in any up-to-date medical author's writings. The medical doctor enters the combat with fear and trembling because he does not know either the cause or the cure.

We will begin by giving our attention to the venous system and the obstruction existing there, resulting in retention, irritation, fermentation, inflammation and gangrene. These are effects. The question is, what cause is responsible for their appearance? We find contraction of the skin, the fascia and the lymphatics obstructing thereby all of the blood and nerve supply of the throat and neck. This contraction extends from the occiput to the diaphragm. We find all of the muscles from the base of the brain to the lower end of the sternum in a state of heavy contraction. We find increased arterial action; also an increased action of the lungs. From the diaphragm upwards we find the arterial supply to be greater than the venous return. Thus we have a mechanical cause that the reason will accept for the retention of blood in all of the glandular systems of the neck and head and their organs. I have found the collar bone with the sternum drawn heavily backwards toward the spine and shutting off the return of blood from the thyroid and other glands of the neck even as high as the occiput.

Prognosis.—The prognosis in diphtheria, as based upon my experience since the application of the principles of osteopathy, is favorable, and I can say to you that my treatment as I give it to you has always been successful when I was called to the patient within reasonable time. When I was not called until high grades of inflammation and gangrene had set in I could relieve the child's suffering to some extent, and even in that condition recovery of my patient occurred, for I cannot remember that I have ever lost a patient suffering with diphtheria since the discovery of osteopathy.

Examination.—Examine carefully your diphtheritic patient, going first to the clavicles and sternum; note their condition then look after the upper ribs, the upper dorsal and cervical vertebrae. See that the cranium articulates normally with the atlas. Examine the hyoid and inferior maxillary bones. Search out the contracted muscles and the cause of their contraction. Know the channels of your blood supply which pass up through the structures of the neck into the cranium and return therefrom, also your nerve supply in the neck.

Never stop in your examination till you have found and taken off the obstruction to the normal supply of blood, nerve and lymph to the structures, then make sure of a thorough and perfect drainage. Examine and know the condition of the kidneys and the bladder. Know that the ureters are freed from all obstructions by pressure or otherwise and are carrying out their normal functions.

Treatment.—In treating a diphtheritic patient I proceed at once to bring the clavicles and sternum far enough forward to take off any pressure that exists, in order to let venous blood and other fluids return to the heart. As I stand back of the patient I place the flat of the fingers of one hand on the front side of the patient's neck in the region of the transverse processes of the atlas and axis. Then with my other hand under the chin I draw it gently forward while holding back on the transverse processes. I draw the chin far enough forward to allow the blood and lymph to pass freely to and from the head, face and neck making sure of perfect drainage down into the innominate veins, thence to the superior vena cava and into the right auricle.

By such work I always get good results when good venous drainage has been secured. I generally bring my fingers with a light flat pressure high up under the jaw in the region of the tonsils. I am careful to adjust from the first to the fourth rib on both sides, then with the child on my lap sitting with its face forward I place my hands flat down on the lower part of the abdomen in the region of the symphysis and make firm gentle pressure there with the flat of my hands, holding awhile then continuing the pressure, I move my hands along the course of the ureters up toward the kidneys, in order to relax all constrictions which exist in that region.

Thus I have prepared the way for the kidneys to deliver urine which generally begins to flow in abundance directly after making the pressure as I have indicated. In a great majority of cases I have found the circulation of the abdomen restored and sweat will break out over it. The fever goes down and the child begins to have rest and natural breathing. I have no use for the usual so-called throat washes, except those required for absolute cleanliness and then the good wholesome gruels. As to hygiene and diet, my advice to mothers has been to practice cleanliness. Give the patient a good clean bed, plenty of fresh air and good nourishing gruels and soups and easily digested foods. The osteopath is to keep close watch over these little patients and treat them two or three times daily, if necessary, according to the severity of the case.

INFLUENZA.

Definition.—Epidemic catarrh; grip or grippe. Severe form of catarrh, usually with marked constitutional symptoms, as great prostration, chills, excessive secretion from nose, larynx, and bronchial tubes, cough, headache, fever, cardiac oppression, etc. The disease is due to infection by a minute organism, the Pfeiffer bacillus or Bacillus influenza. It usually occurs epidemically, and generally affects a large number of persons in a community. Its duration is from a few days to a week or more. It occurs under three main forms, the cerebral, gastroenteric, and pulmonary, named from the systems most severely attacked.

—Dunglison.

Etiology.—The up-to-date medical books give the same old theories which can be found throughout all the medical world as to the cause of influenza. In our discussion of this condition we will lay aside all of the "pathies" with their many theories and take up the matter as a mechanic would take up the machinery with which he is familiar and which is out of repair and ask as he would ask: "What is the matter with the machine? Why will it not do its work as it was intended it should?"

In making your examination of these patients who are suffering with influenza, La Grippe, catarrhal fever, or bad cold (call it what you will) you will find them in a state of general muscular contraction due to atmospheric changes.

Prognosis.—The osteopathic prognosis for speedy relief of influenza is good when the osteopath has been called to the case within any reasonable time.

Examination.—As I have hinted at muscular contraction I will now try to point out to the operator the territory in which during many years of practice I have found rigidity. It includes all the muscles of the neck, the trachea and the esophagus, also the heavy contractions of the spinal and intercostal muscles extending as low down as the diaphragm. This exploration is to cover all the region from the ninth rib up on each side of the spine.

I carefully examine all ribs from the ninth to the first for the least variation from the truly normal articulation, and know that every rib is in its proper

292

position both on the sternum and in its spinal articulations. I make this examination thorough because the rigidity of the spinal and cervical muscles while under the spasmodic action of a heavy cold brings the ribs so close together as to interfere with the blood and nerve supply to the entire thoracic system.

Treatment.—When treating my influenza patients I generally stand in front of them, be they old or young, and have them place their arms on my shoulders, then I begin to explore from about the tenth rib upwards. I carefully examine the ribs of both sides as I go up to ascertain whether the rib is pulled down below the transverse process of the spine or is pushed up above it. When I find it displaced either way I halt right there and adjust that rib. I then continue, adjusting everything found out of line as I go up until I get to the first rib. I then make sure whether or not the clavicle is drawn heavily against the anterior surface of the neck; whether the clavicle, the first or second rib is pulled down and back and producing a compression of the inferior cervical ganglion. This I consider of the greatest importance because right here we will find, if we reason at all, a weight or pressure irritating the nervous system that governs the arterial supply and the venous drainage.

When I have adjusted all structures and obtained the truly normal condition of this portion of the thorax I have looked for and have obtained early relief in all cases. This irritation will stimulate the arterial system to a higher grade of action and will impede or stop the drainage of venous and other fluids that should be carried without hindrance back to the heart. I continue my explorations through the entire length of the neck from its articulation with the dorsal vertebrae on up to the occiput. I have often found the atlas drawn forward and almost closing the space between itself and the inferior maxilla. This should be carefully and properly adjusted before relief may be expected by him who reasons as a mechanic.

By the obstructions indicated here I have satisfied my mind as a mechanic that herein lies the cause in this disease of the disturbance of the stomach, the heart, the lung and the other organs above the diaphragm. I will advise the operator first, last and all the time to read and review the nerve and blood supply from the latest and best anatomical authors so as to have fresh in your mind the entire circulation to the parts affected. Herein lies your hope. I fully agree with the medical doctor who says that drugs avail but little, if any, as

293

remedies in such conditions. Remove the obstruction, restore the circulation to and from the parts and your work is done and you have your reward.

As to nursing and dieting I have generally advised the patient to take swallows of warm soup often through the day and night, my object being to lubricate the mouth and pharynx. I use no washes or gargles more than to let my patients drink all the water they want and when they feel like it. In regard to the temperature of the room and fresh air I instruct that the room and bedding should be kept so as to permit the patient to feel comfortable.

ERYSIPELAS.

Definition.—St. Anthony's fire, wildfire. A disease characterized by superficial inflammation of the skin, with general fever, tension, and swelling of the part; the surface is smooth and shining, as if oiled; pain and heat, redness diffuse, but more or less circumscribed, and disappearing when pressed upon by the finger, but returning as soon as the pressure is removed. Frequently small vesicles appear upon the inflamed part, which dry up and fall off as branny scales. This disease is contagious and inoculable, and is thought to be the result of the introduction of the Streptococcus erysipelatis or erysipelatos.
—*Dunglison.*

Etiology.—I am satisfied from long experience in handling erysipelas that the cause of this malady is venous blood obstructed and held in the parts affected long enough for inflammation and decomposition to take place. When the case is one of the facial types, which is the most common, then I generally find trouble with the articulations of the inferior maxilla, the cervical vertebrae, the clavicles or the upper ribs. These bones are out of their normal positions and pressing upon some of the vessels of the neck. I also find contractured muscles under the angle and back of the jaw obstructing the jugular veins and pressing upon the superior cervical ganglion.

Treatment.—When I have been called upon to treat facial erysipelas I have used the following method. With my patient sitting erect on a chair or stool I stand at the side, place the fingers of one hand behind the angle of the jaw and those of the other against the transverse processes of the upper cervical vertebrae, the atlas and axis in particular, and with my breast I bear down on the head with light pressure while at the same time I gently but firmly pull the jaw forward and away from the neck. I do this to open up the structures and especially to loosen up the muscles surrounding the vessels through which the venous blood must pass on its way back to the heart. Then I change sides and go through the same process on the other side of the head and neck.

I make sure that the hyoid bone is not drawn to one side by muscular contracture and impinging on any vessels or nerves. I open the blood-vessels of the axilla on both sides of the body by simply reaching one hand over the patient's breast the other over the back, opposite to the side where I stand and meet or bring them together in the axilla. Then gently but firmly pull the arm and muscles up and thoroughly loosen them.

I adjust carefully both collar bones to their normal positions after the method which I have given you for their adjustment in the treatment of measles, small pox, and so on. Be patient, take plenty of time for your work, and rest not until you have made the drainage of the facial veins a certainty. Be very careful that you have adjusted the inferior maxilla because it is very often quite out of its normal position. In some cases this is the result of dental work. After the extraction of teeth the under jaw has been left in a strained position.

When the case is severe the treatment is to be given once, twice or even three times the first day. But my object has never been the number of treatments but the certainty of drainage which is always accompanied in a short time by a disappearance of the fever, swelling, soreness and all other distressing symptoms.

The treatment should be followed up till satisfactory results are secured and recovery is complete. The light in the room is to be gauged by the wishes of the patient. So also the bed as to its being hard or soft. Good plain nutritious food is to be given. Keep all outward applications off of the face. Dry cotton bound on the face with a handkerchief or other cloth is all the dressing I ever found necessary.

Erysipelas of the arm, leg, chest or any portion of the body I treat following the same principle, proceeding as quickly as possible to establish natural drainage of the venous blood in that portion of the body which is affected. Know your descriptive anatomy in order to keep the nerve and blood systems constantly before your eyes when combating erysipelas.

As a precaution against constipation and kidney trouble I carefully examine the splanchnic area, also the renal, and adjust any vertebrae or ribs that are found out of their normal positions.

MUMPS.

Definition.—Contagious parotiditis; a contagious febrile disease marked by inflammation and swelling of the parotid gland. After an incubation-period of about three weeks the symptoms appear with fever, headache, and pain beneath the ear. Soon there develops a tense, painful swelling in the parotid region, which interferes with mastication and swallowing and renders both actions painful. After a period of a few days to a week the symptoms gradually disappear. Sometimes the submaxillary and other salivary glands are involved, and occasionally the testicles, mammae, or the labia majora become swollen. One attack generally confers immunity from another.

—Dorland.

Etiology.—Mumps is a contagious disease. While it is not known what it is or how it gets into the system, there is known something of its effects. We know that the glands of the neck high up as well as those of the face swell and impede and irritate the natural action of arterial blood in its passage from the heart through the neck into the head as well as the venous return.

The anatomist is well acquainted with these facts. He knows also the nerve supply and that it cannot do normal work when impinged. He knows that both in the male and the female patient the normal action of the salivary glands, the lymphatics and all of the generative system of glands as well as the excretory glands is suspended by the workings of this disease which is called mumps, and which would be just as well expressed if it were called lumps.

Our business is to know where the obstruction is and then to remove it giving the blood and all other fluids that are thereby hindered in their normal circulation or channels of action a chance to go on normally. The result is a disappearance of the fever, reduction of the glandular enlargement of the neck, free action of the kidneys and relief for the ovaries in the female and testicles in the male.

Treatment.—Your work begins with the neck at its union with the head. Make sure you adjust any ah normality existing there. Use close observation and carefully adjust every bone of the neck from the atlas on down; every rib from the first to the twelfth; also both clavicles. Do all this work carefully and thoroughly. Then adjust your structures from the tenth dorsal to the sacrum because here you will find obstructive congestion. See that the eleventh and twelfth ribs are raised and in normal articulation with their vertebrae. Secure perfect adjustment of the lumbar vertebrae.

I will speak of one way whereby the vertebrae of the lumbar region may be adjusted. If your patient be an adult male or female and sufficiently well to be out of bed, stand him in the doorway with his face and breast against the jamb of the door, then bring a gentle but firm pressure with your knee at the upper part of the sacrum and with your hands on both his shoulders pull his body back far enough to bring gentle pressure over your knee, then swing him from right to left a few times so as to thoroughly loosen up the lumbar region.

When your patient is on his back inhibit the occipital nerves to loosen the musculature then carefully loosen and adjust both atlas and axis. Take the patient's chin in one hand the occiput in the other and pull the chin gently forward and up to loosen the muscles of the neck. Now go to the symphysis and with a gentle and firm pressure hold a little, then bring the hands slowly and firmly toward the kidneys over the region of the ureters. Now the bladder is ready to receive and you have the excretory system ready to act in its function of carrying off the waste products of the body.

Let your patient lie on his back in a comfortable room for a few days. Such good plain nutritious food as the patient's appetite calls for can be given. This has been my practice and experience for many years and has been successful ln all cases without exception.

CHICKENPOX.

Definition of Varicella.—Chickenpox. A disease characterized by vesicles scattered over the body, which are glabrous, transparent, and about the size of peas. They appear in successive crops, are covered by a thin pellicle, and about the third, fourth, or fifth day from their appearance burst at the top and concrete into small, puckered scabs, which rarely leave a pit in the skin.

—Dunglison.

Etiology.—Chickenpox does its work more on the nutrient system and the sweat glands of the skin than elsewhere. Thus we find reason to look for pressure on the nutrient nerves of the skin beginning high up and in front of the neck and back of the jaw. There we will find trouble. In that space where the cervical arteries enter the head we will find a bulky or a piled up condition of the muscles. We also find heavy pressure of bones and muscles on the blood-vessels as they pass under the clavicles and upper ribs back to the vena cava. Here we have a cause that produces the effect called chickenpox. By shutting off or impeding the blood and nerve supply to the sweat glands of the skin there is a shock to the brain, the lungs, the heart, the nutrient and the entire excretory system of the skin.

Treatment.—In a general way treat this effect according to the method given you under the heading of smallpox. Be very careful and very thorough in your neck adjustments. Loosen the atlas and axis and draw forward the inferior maxilla from its pressure upon the vessels and nerves back of its angle. Draw the hyoid bone forward and secure good circulation of blood throughout the entire cervical region.

SMALLPOX.

Definition of Variola.—Smallpox. Very contagious disease, characterized by fever, pain in the back, vomiting, and an eruption of papules, appearing from the third to the fifth day, and suppurating from the eighth to the tenth. The disease possesses all the distinctive properties of the major exanthemata. It is capable of being produced by inoculation, but this inoculated smallpox—variola inserta—communicates the disease as readily through the air as the natural smallpox, or that received without inoculation. Smallpox is divided into two classes, according to the character of the eruption—the discrete or distinct and the confluent: 1. In variola discreta, distinct smallpox, the pustules are usually the size of peas, distinct, distended, and circular, the intervening spaces being red the fever inflammatory throughout, and ceasing when the eruption is complete. 2. In variola confluens, confluent smallpox, the pustules are confluent or run together; flaccid and irregularly circumscribe, the intervening spaces being pale, and the accompanying fever typhoid in character. In children diarrhoea, and in adults ptyalism, with swelling of the hands and feet, generally appear toward the stage of the secondary fever, which occurs from the tenth to the thirteenth day. The fever that precedes and accompanies the eruption is called the eruptive fever. The prognosis is ordinarily favorable in the discrete variety. The confluent is always dangerous, the unfavorable symptoms being flattening of the pustules or subsidence of the eruption, the breathing becoming much obstructed or oppressed, or marks of inflammatory and congestive affections occurring in the different viscera. When the pimples are confluent in patches, the patches being, however, separated by intervals of unaffected skin, it constitutes the clustered, coherent, or corymbose variety—variola corymbosa. When there are comparatively few pustules, and the general eruption scarcely passes beyond the vesicular stage, the term varicelloid smallpox, variola curta, varioloid, has been applied to it. Other forms of variola have been mentioned, such as the petechial and hemorrhagic, variola cruenta, or black pox, variola gangroenosa, etc.

—*Dunglison.*

Etiology.—I reason that the effect we see in small pox follows the stoppage of watery substances in the superficial fascia. Smallpox does its work in the superficial and deep fascias of the whole system. Heavy contractions of muscles and ligaments overcome the normal action of the excretory system of the whole body and this results in congestion, stagnation, decom position and pus formation in the deep and superficial fascias.

The only method by which the superficial fascia can rid itself of its load is to pass the diseased substances through the skin by boring a sufficient number of holes and so making a passage out for the dead fluids which fester as they go. Thus we have a cause for the great number of large and small boils or pocks, and by this method of reasoning I have tried to draw the attention of the osteopath to the part of the body in which small pox proceeds to do its destructive work of obstructing the normal circulation of blood and other fluids under and through the skin. The effect that we see follows the stoppage of the watery substances in the superficial fascia and is what is known as smallpox contagion. In my experience I have found at the upper part of the neck a thickening of the muscles which unite it to the base of the skull. I have always found enlargement and contracture of muscles, ligaments and tissues in the region of the openings into the skull through which the carotid and vertebral arteries pass to convey blood into the brain. I have found a great deal of spasmodic contraction that would excite arterial action above the normal. I have also found almost a complete obstruction of the venous return through this locality due to the contraction above described. I think this contraction causes very much of this arterial blood to be forced into and retained in the glandular system of the neck, face and head, and results in the enlargement of these glands of the heck. I think this process overcomes the entire nerve supply of the whole lymphatic system and all of its organs. This spasmodic contraction at the union of the neck with the head I find to be strong enough to move the atlas either laterally, anteriorly or posteriorly as I have invariably found it displaced when called to treat smallpox patients.

Treatment.—As a mechanic I approach the engine of life and begin my examination at the occiput. If I find any variation of the atlas or axis forward, backward, to the right or to the left, I proceed at once to adjust them to their normal places in order to let the venous blood out of the head and also to free up the whole pneumogastric system. Now as the contraction extends down

301

the neck and the venous blood has to be delivered into the innominate veins I proceed to adjust and loosen up the clavicles and the upper four ribs on both sides of the spine. I do this in order to take any pressure by bone or muscle off the descending jugulars and to keep the road open the entire course from the occiput to the heart. Then I proceed to carefully examine the next four ribs on both sides because I want the intercostal arteries and veins of the thorax above the diaphragm to be absolutely free, and the flow of arterial and venous blood unobstructed. After this I proceed to adjust all ribs below those designated and all spinal articulations, in order to secure normal action of the kidneys and of the entire excretory system which has been suspended by contraction in some part.

I place my hands just above the symphysis making a flat strong pressure while I draw my fingers along the region of the ureters and on up to the kidneys with the view of giving freedom to the flow of urine from the kidneys down to the bladder. When there is much headache I inhibit the occipital nerves that pass out and up over the atlas. In adjusting the bones of the neck and back of my smallpox patients, I treat them in the bed letting the patient be on his back. I spread the arms straight out from the body one at a time. Then I pull the collar bone to its place. I also reach over the shoulder and catch the upper ribs and pull them forward as I have explained before. I treat these patients from one to three times a day until relief is given. Be careful to use no severe treatment in adjusting any of these bones. This would do more harm than good. Inasmuch as these patients come under the laws of quarantine and isolation I will say my rule has been to obey the laws. I have the room reasonably well darkened. As to diet I have been governed by reason and advise the individual accordingly. Give a diet reason able in quantity and quality. I have the sheets and bedding changed according to my own judgment and the circumstances surrounding each individual case. None of my patients and so far as I know none of the patients of other osteopaths have died of smallpox.

SMALLPOX PREVENTED BY A HARMLESS GERMIFUGE.

[With a few slight changes this article is as it appeared in the January (1902) number of the Journal of Osteopathy.]

In cantharidin commonly known as the Spanish fly, my mother discovered a perfectly harmless and effective germifuge. During the past few years I have subjected it to every possible test in all parts of the United States where smallpox has been rampant. I have never found a single instance in which the trial has not proven my claim that cantharidin will immune man from smallpox without harmful results. Many are familiar with the results obtained in Kirksville during our recent so-designated "smallpox scare." We used it on from 2000 to 2500 of our townspeople with unquestionable results.

All these years Jenner's discovery has been the single weapon wielded by the medical profession in the fight against the dreaded disease so far as a germifuge was used in the battle. Notwithstanding that the so-called preventative has in thousands upon thousands of cases proven worse than the disease smallpox itself, the doctors have been content to follow Jenner's teachings. There is no evidence on record that any effort has ever been made to effect a departure from the long taught and faithfully practiced lesson of injecting the cowpox virus with its hidden impurities into the arm of man to immune him from smallpox.

For centuries the subject of smallpox has been a serious one for the minds and pens of the doctors. From them we have learned nothing of the origin nor of the action of the deadly poison which it contains. When we sum up all that has been written we only learn that the doctor does not know what it is or what it does except to kill millions of the human race. Concerning smallpox our wisest doctors know nothing more than the savage with no books. So in the twentieth century we need not look backward for knowledge on this subject. For the doctors the field is just as cloudy today as in the period of the remotest days of man's history when he thought that God had sent smallpox as one of his choicest plagues to punish the nations for some sin of disobedience to His holy ordinance. Man has tried many things to stop the deadly work of smallpox; he has prayed, sacrificed and dosed, but to no effect.

My first experience with smallpox was in Kansas where I was associated early in my practice of medicine with my father who also was a disciple of the "old school." About the time that Kansas was opened to settlement, smallpox and all other eruptive fevers began to make their appearance and do their deadly work. Of all diseases man is heir to, I dreaded smallpox the most, for if it did not kill it left one disfigured for life. I had been vaccinated a great number of times but without effect, and I felt then that should I contract the disease I would have little hope of living through it. Thus smallpox was my dread by day and by night.

A number of times I was called to a case not knowing it was smallpox until after entering the house. It was then too late to back down and I had to submit to the inevitable. Frequently I had well developed cases of confluent smallpox to treat and I generally got my patient through safely. Later I was called to a supposed case of fever which proved to be confluent small pox from which the man died. His wife had a sore eye and upon examining it I was surprised to find a pock of variola with which she had suffered many days. It was from that pock her husband had taken the contagion and died. Again I was in fear and agony that from that family I would contract the disease and die for I had no vaccine pock mark to hold between myself and the dreaded coffin.

At this time (1862) my anxiety was intellectually and very satisfactorily modified by a conversation with my mother. She said that possibly while a boy I had absorbed enough of the fly-blister which she had applied to my hip for a case of white swelling, as she then called it, to perhaps make me immune from smallpox. She had blistered and reblistered my hip for three months. During this process many pieces of bone came out of the crest of the ilium, and the marks are abundant today, both of the ulcers and the blisters. I have long since come to the conclusion that the cantharidin thus absorbed was the cause of the immunity that stood between me and the smallpox. I am also convinced that the cause of unsuccessful vaccination, the cowpox virus having been often inserted into my arm from childhood up to manhood and without effect, was the cantharidin in my system. For the discovery of this I give credit to my mother, Martha P. Still, Centropolis, Kansas. After forty years of convincing experience I have concluded to give the world the benefit of it.

I would not antagonize the popular belief in the efficacy of vaccination but do most emphatically combat the insertion into the human body of putrid flesh of any animal. With this belief in reference to vaccination as a preventative of smallpox and with the chances to contract other diseases to which the cow and horse are subject so very possible and well proven by the great number of persons who have been vaccinated and crippled for life, I concluded that it was about time for the sons and daughters of America to take up the subject of prevention and see how their skill would compare with that of Jenner of England. In the January (1901) number of the Journal of Osteopathy I published an article discussing the probable value of cantharidin as one of the greatest germifuges of the world.

A Spanish fly-blister about the size of a dollar when placed upon the arm above the elbow will at once start an infectious fever whose energy is in full eruptive blast in from four to six hours, or forty-eight times faster than variola which requires twelve days to reach its highest energy. My philosophy is that the first infectious fever that is an active occupant of the body will drive off others and hold possession of the body until its power is spent and the excretory system has renovated the body. The possession of the human body by an infectious germ can only immune by germicidal possession. In this way we are immune by vaccination or any other infectious substance while it is in possession of and effecting the machinery of human vitality, and no longer. According to its friends and advocates the effect of vaccination leaves the body in from one to seven years and then there is a demand for repeated vaccination with its lurking dangers. A Spanish fly-blister may be used on the arm many times a year if necessary and act as a preventing germifuge without harm.

I have solicited correspondence from doctors of sixty years of age and upwards, on the subject of the fly blister's work in their early practice when it was used in any and all forms of disease. The correspondence has been exceedingly gratifying to me for in every instance where my correspondent could correctly answer my questions, my deductions as to the value of cantharidin as a germifuge in smallpox have been sustained. But what is more to the point, since my article appeared in the Journal of Osteopathy last January the graduates of the American School of Osteopathy, who have been guided by my instruction, have reported thousands upon thousands of cases in which cantharidin had been used as a preventative of smallpox during an epidemic and not a single individual whose arm had been blistered as directed contracted the disease.

I have often been asked, what are my ideas of vaccination. I have no use for it at all nor any faith in it since witnessing its slaughterous work. It slew our armies in the sixties and is still torturing our old soldiers, not to say anything of its more recent victims whose number will run up into tens upon tens of thousands. I believe that instead of passing laws for compulsory vaccination, a law prohibiting the practice and providing heavy penalties for violations would prove a wholesome experiment. Take the fifty cents out of the "dirty" practice and it will die out spontaneously with all doctors of average knowledge of the harm done by it. The philosopher must find something better as a germifuge, or by legal measures, hands off. I have long believed that the wisdom of man was sufficient for a successful hunt for an innocent and trustworthy germifuge for smallpox, and that it would be found early in the twentieth century if we would but work and reason.

I will not dispute or try to criticise so great a man as Jenner, but I will say that in all the histories of the man and in his own works I do not find a single word of his philosophy nor any reason why he believed that the cowpox would fortify the human body against the entry of smallpox. He simply reported that a less number of milkers took the smallpox after they had "sore hands" supposed to have been caused by getting the poison in some cut, scratch or broken surface of the skin of the hands. Since his day the world has been content to hunt for that "stuff" that was on the cow's udder. No questions were asked, it was simply, "I want some of that stuff what makes folks hands git sore." Jenner did put "rot" into his patients to keep the "rot" of smallpox out, so you see there was a fight for possession between the two great "rots" and the cow-rot is supposed to have hooked off the smallpox rot. That is all the immunity there is about cowpox holding free from smallpox.

I believe that the discovery of Jenner gave nothing to the world excepting the history of an accidental cure or supposed preventative to smallpox. He gave no reason why one poison would immune the person from another poison. The doctors simply accepted, tried and adopted the supposed remedial power of cowpox, sore or cankered heels of the horse. They gave us no caution or hint that the grease heels of the horse might be a venereal disease peculiar to the horse only. They told us nothing of the cowpox, whether or not it was venereal in its nature. Like the adoption of most "remedies" the doctor uses or has used, it came to notice by accident.

I do not wish in the least to antagonize the efforts of Jenner. His efforts were good, but more effective and less dangerous substances can be used than the putrid compounds of variola. I believe that cantharidin will be found just as protective against measles, diphtheria, scarlet fever, leprosy and syphilis and other infectious contagions as against smallpox. This is the twentieth century and our school was created to improve on past methods and theories let us keep step with the music of progress. I feel certain that the time is close at hand when compulsory vaccination will not be necessary, for a better method, one that will do the work and leave no bad effects as is the case in vaccination with the cow, horse or other animal poisons, has been found. The dread of disease and death that follow vaccination causes people to hesitate before having vaccine matter put into their own arms or into the arms of their children by military force. When they learn that a fly-blister as large as a fifty-cent piece or a dollar will keep off smallpox in all cases, then there will be no fear or trouble about smallpox or vaccination.

HOW TO USE FLY-BLISTER.

For an adult, take an amount of fly-blister equal to the size of two grains of corn. Spread it smoothly over a piece of coarse sheeting two inches square so it will cover the cloth. After washing the arm clean, put the plaster on it nearer the shoulder than the elbow avoiding old vaccine scars. When the skin looks quite red take off the plaster and dress it with dry cotton. Allow this dressing to remain until the arm itches. Then take off the dressing if the cotton is loose. If not loose leave it on the arm a day or two to allow the blistered spot to heal. The work is then all done. For a child under ten years of age, use a plaster about one inch square. Do not have a plaster on an infant over an hour before examination, and when it is quite red take it off and dress it with dry cotton without washing. Do not use oils of any kind as a dressing. Watch carefully and do not blister too deep. A single blister will immune for a long time, but it is well enough when a heavy epidemic appears to blister the arm again. There is not a shadow of danger from its use. The power of cantharidin as a germifuge has been proven but it is important that only pure fly-blister be used.

CHOLERA.

Definition.—An acute, infectious disease, of very rapid course, endemic in certain parts of India and making occasional epidemic incursions into other countries. In a typical case there are three stages: first, of diarrhea; second, of rice-water evacuations, vomiting, cramps, coldness and lividity of the skin, etc., with a peculiar pinched expression of the face and collapse; and a third stage, in favorable cases, of reaction or consecutive fever. In temperate climates common cholera is not usually a disease of much consequence.

—*Dunglison.*

Description and Symptoms.—I will give the reader the benefit of my personal experience with that dreadful disease, cholera. In 1852 while I was living in Macon County, Mo., it broke out among my neighbors, several of whom died from its ravages. One brother was attacked with it and it came very near taking him off. During that year it was very prevalent throughout the United States and there were many cases in Missouri and Kansas. Being at that time in the practice of medicine I was called to treat many of these cases.

I do not know what cholera is, whence it came nor whither it went. I know that during its prevalence in Missouri and previous to this time there had been a very wet season, an unusually heavy rainfall followed by chilly, cold spring weather, then the sudden appearance of hot days and the cholera began to spread. It generally began with sickness at the stomach, followed by vomiting and purging which would continue a few hours. There was little headache. The eyes were glassy and sunken. The pulse was slow. The lungs were also slow in action. When air was inhaled it seemed as though the lungs could not possibly be satisfied notwithstanding enough atmosphere had been taken in to raise the chest abnormally high. When the air was exhaled the ribs and sternum seemed to shrink back to an abnormal drawing in of the entire chest. I think that four to six inhalations to the minute was about the velocity of the lung action. The patients had a peculiar groan which I will describe as a long Oh! Soon after this groaning began, the perspiration broke out all over the body even as though it were a sponge full of water. On every inhalation the entire porus system poured out water until I have seen it run through sheet, mattress, and across the floor and escape through the cracks. I think that the water leaving the body at this stage all brought together would have made up a continuous stream as large as an ordinary round lead pencil.

I was called to a patient, a Mrs. Pierce who lived six or eight miles in the country. She was dead when I reached the house. They told me of the intensity of her suffering and of the dreadful cramps. On examination I found her hip drawn clear out of the acetabulum and it was necessary to adjust it before she could be placed in the coffin. I heard of others with spasms as severe but this was the only case which came directly under my notice. What peculiar condition the atmosphere gets into to produce this deadly effect I do not know.

During 1854 and '55 I was in Kansas and had a more extended experience with cholera and was very familiar with its progress and the popular method of treating it which proved quite successful. Its onset was so sudden that people prepared and kept in the house a compound which they called cholera medicine. It was composed of a quart of whisky, two ounces of tincture gum kino, one ounce of tincture capsicum and one quarter of an ounce of opium. They took a quarter of a tumbler of this every three hours until relief came. At this time I knew nothing of osteopathy and the dependence of all was upon drugs. Since that time I have only met with severe cases of cholera morbus which were to all appearances cholera, having all its symptoms. This in every case readily yielded to osteopathic treatment.

Etiology.—With my experience to this day as a medical doctor and an osteopathic mechanic I have reasoned about and located the beginning of the cholera attack in the lungs. I have observed this, that the entire chest, both back and front is very cold. In the fifties I had not thought of the cold chest or the cold body being in the state that the hydrogen and the oxygen would con dense into water while in the lungs. When I saw the streams of water leaving the body my thought was simply, that this was a case of cholera. I was young, and no author nor council with whom I met ever suggested to me the fact that the lungs could generate and the body absorb water enough to drown out all the nutrient principles of the blood. A few years later I reasoned that hydrogen and oxygen would condense on a bottle and prove that these two gases produced water. To confirm this conclusion I remembered the effect of the home-made cholera medicine, the compound of whisky, capsicum, gum kino and opium as it was given to those patients who were not too far gone, how it warmed them up and how they got well.

At that time I did not reason that a low body temperature preceded the exhausting sweats of cholera, neither did I reason that a high temperature of the body would stop the process. I did not reason that the atmospheric air when taken into the lungs formed a union of hydrogen, oxygen and other gases, forming water which would be taken up by the entire secretory system and be distributed throughout the body until it had complete watery possession; as much so as the equivalent bulk of water, which a sponge will take up and which by squeezing may be expressed like the great perspiration that is seen in cholera. At that time I also learned the wonderful and dangerous effect of fear which I believe was the cause to a great extent of the system being thrown into this water producing and discarding condition.

Let me give you a case to illustrate this question of fear and to give you a word of warning. A young man who was my chum accepted an invitation to accompany me on a visit to my father and mother who in 1854 were living at the Shawnee Mission fifty miles west of Kansas City and close to the Kaw River. We made our visit to the mission and started on our journey back to Macon County, Mo., returning by the way of Kansas City where we heard much talk about the ravages of cholera on the boats and at all the river towns from Kansas City to New Orleans. Cholera was the leading subject of conversation with all persons whom we met as we traveled east. When we were about sixty miles from Kansas City and on the high prairie I felt that we were out of all danger and just like joking, so I told my chum that I had the cholera. I thought nothing of the effect of such a speech but before we had journeyed a quarter of a mile farther he turned as pale as death and showed all the signs of a sudden attack of cholera—perspiration, cold body, nausea and all. At this time I tried to reason with him. I told him that I felt so fine at our escape from the danger I was joking and that I had no cholera. But this had no effect upon him and I was afraid he would die then and there. He paid no attention to anything I said, and to all appearances seemed likely to go into a collapse in a few moments. Not knowing just how to bring him to himself, and remembering what changes would come over me when father would take a strap of leather and strap me all over and how between my anger and the strap my body soon became quite warm, I was not long in coming to a conclusion to strap my friend to bring about the necessary reaction from the fright he was in. So I reached down and loosened my stirrup strap and began to lay it on him heavy. He paid no attention until I had struck him at least a half dozen strokes, then he looked at me and said, "you hurt." He was in his shirt sleeves and I continued to lay the strap across his back good and heavy until his anger was roused and he said, "If you don't quit that I'll knock you off your horse." Then I knew my medicine was taking effect and I was happy to know that my chum would not die there on the open prairie many miles from home.

During the twenty-five years following this occurrence we often met and he always said and stuck to it that the leather strap well laid on to him at that time was what saved his life. This taught me a lesson that I have never forgotten and one that I want to emphasize to every osteopath—never tell a patient that he is in a bad fix, worse today than yesterday, or that he looks ill. I believe more patients suffer and die from such imprudence and fright than the world has ever dreamed of.

Treatment.—Since I have given the description and my philosophy of cholera, I will say that I have never seen a case of Asiatic Cholera since 1855. But I have seen many cases of cholera morbus that were good imitations in every particular of the genuine Asiatic Cholera. There was great suffering in the lumbar region, headache, sickness at stomach, exhausting perspiration and so on. In my treatment of these cases my object was to relieve the spasmodic condition of the muscles of the lumbar region and those of the spine up to the head. If my patient was in bed I had him get out and kneel down at the side of it with his chest resting on the edge of the bed. Then I came up behind him, spread out my knees and took his hips between them. Then with my thumbs one on each side of the spinous processes of the lumbar vertebrae I made hard pressure while with my knees I gave his body an oscillating motion, my aim being to give his hips a twist with my knees while I moved my thumbs from joint to joint as I twisted. I continued this on up to the twelfth dorsal.

Now I have thoroughly loosened up the spine, its muscles and ligaments; and wanting to do the same for the axillary region and its circulation, while in this same position I place my right hand on top of the patient's left shoulder close to the neck and pull down strongly while taking the left arm in my hand I raise it out and up strongly. This will loosen up the axillary nerves and blood-vessels. Now I change sides and put my left hand on the right shoulder, reaching over as far as the clavicle and raising the right arm as I did the left. I now ask my patient to sit on the side of the bed while I inhibit the occipital nerves. While working here I am very careful to know that the atlas is in line and in good articulation.

I follow this process two or three times each day until I know that my work is well done and so proven by the ease and comfort that I have given my patient in place of the great agony and misery which accompany this disease. The results following this method of treatment have always been good. As to nourishment for these patients let it be simple, plain, nutritious soups or gruels. I have hinted here at the philosophy of the cause of cholera and hope and trust that others will prosecute the subject further.

MALARIA.

Definition.—A febrile disease due to the presence in the red blood corpuscles of an animal microparasite, the Plasmodium malariae. Marchiafava and Bignami distinguish three forms of malaria, each having its peculiar parasite: quartan, tertian, aestivo-autumnal. The infection occurs through the bite of the mosquito (Anopheles), which has herself been infected by previously drawing blood from a person suffering from malaria. The sovereign remedy for malaria is quinine. Chronic malaria leads to a condition called malarial cachexia, marked by impoverishment of the blood, enlargement of the spleen, and an earthy color of the skin.

—Abbreviated from *Dunglison*.

Etiology.—I have given you Dunglison's short definition, and according to my opinion a shorter definition of the same kind by Dunglison would have been just as good. I have spent over fifty years north of 36 and south of 46 degrees north latitude and in my youth I had the fever and ague or malaria three or four times. In the latitudes 40 to 44 degrees north we observe chills and fever generally occurring during the latter days of August and on through the month of September because about that time the sun recedes to the south and the direction of the rays of heat change becoming less perpendicular. For several weeks the heat of the sun ranging from 90 to 110 degrees is being poured upon the human body during those long days and this I think so far exhausts the nerves of the spine that they become relaxed and give way. This is the effect of the long continued heat especially upon those whose business requires them to be much of the time in the sun or exposed to its rays. They fall upon or are reflected upon buildings having much southern exposure to the sun where clerks must work by windows for long hours. Men and children are most liable to malaria. No age is exempt from it. Carpenters, railroad workers, sewer and ditch diggers are among those exposed to and are the persons whom I have observed are affected at this season of the year with malaria. Grandma never had it because she kept in the shade. The doctor seldom had it because in riding horseback in his country practice he usually rode under the shade of the umbrella.

313

Merchants, blacksmiths and others whose business keeps them in the shade seldom have chills and fever. Carpenters in a new country very often have malaria because they are much exposed to the rays of the sun directly on their backs while at work on houses.

I will say that from my observation in proportion to the improvement in buildings, the growth of shade trees, and the use of buggy tops and umbrellas to intercept the direct rays of the sun from falling on those persons living between 36 and 46 degrees north latitude, together with the sanitation, improved diet and conveniences that multiply with the age of a new country, malaria disappears. As to the mosquito being the doctor's vaccinator of malarial poisons such philosophy and reasoning is not accepted as a demonstrated fact in this latitude. Between 26 and 36 degrees north latitude bilious fevers prevail with greater severity. Whether the yellow fever gets in its work between the equator and 26 degrees north latitude because of the mosquito or the filthy gas arising from unsanitary closets, stagnant water or decaying vegetation is a question, as this fever seems to disappear when the order for cleanliness is enforced in a city.

I will spend no further time theorizing on supposable causes and will now give my attention to the cry of the sick person who is called upon to suffer with chills and fever for one to three days each week, and who has prescribed for him one to ten doses of calomel, blue mass and other mercurial preparations, castor oil, and quinine as a sovereign remedy, without relief from those periodical spells of torment. The first question I ask my patient is: Does your back ache before the chill comes on? The answer universally is, "yes." Where does it hurt you the most? Answer is, "the small of my back," the hands being placed on the lumbar region say from the tenth dorsal on down to the sacrum. Do you have any headache? "Yes, right after my chill I have severe headache." How else are you troubled? "I am sick at my stomach, sometimes I vomit." How were your bowels before you took down? "They were very, very loose, a good deal of running off with some blood for two or three weeks before the chills came on." Do you pass much urine? "No, and what I do pass is very dark and brownish in its color."

Treatment.—The treatment which I have used successfully for thirty-five years in chills and fever of malaria has been to adjust the lumbar vertebrae which are humped up and posterior almost making a rainbow in shape. When

314

the patient is a man I generally treat him in the lumbar region while he is standing up, placing him with his face and breast against the jamb of a door. I set my knee on the upper part of the sacrum, hold that firmly then place my hands on his shoulders. I draw him backwards then make a few moves to the right and the left in order to adjust the sacrum to its normal articulation and take the pressure off the renal system.

After this I set my patient on an ordinary chair and stand in front of him then I pass my hand under his arms clear back to the spinous processes in the region of the eighth dorsal vertebra. While in that position I pull that part of the body up and toward me and continue this work up the dorsal region till I know that the vertebrae are all in correct line and the ribs in their natural articulations. I adjust all the bones of the neck because I wish to relieve the congestion of the cerebellum, medulla and all the nerves above the diaphragm.

Now I lay both hands on the lower abdomen with my fingers touching the symphysis. I make a heavy, firm pressure and draw my hands up in a line to the kidneys. Right here I want to emphasize that you are to do no gouging with the points of your fingers. By so doing you are liable to do some serious injury. Gentle pressure and no gouging when treating the abdomen of a patient for any purpose whatsoever. I give this precaution knowing that occasionally some persons use much force without thought or caution. You may by foolish gouging produce a wound or injury to the omentum, peritoneum, liver, kidney, spleen or any other abdominal organ or structure, hence be careful.

The ordinary plain nutritious food is good enough. As a general thing malarial patients have a very poor appetite. With this system of treating I have had complete success, recovery following in all cases in a very few days and improvement taking place from the very hour of the first treatment. I treat once or twice a day at first, then I have my patient come to me about twice a week. This I have found to be sufficient.

From my observation for many years I have come to the conclusion that the condition known as malaria is an effect which follows such a general contraction of the structures of the body as will interfere with the entire excretory system and this general contraction can be relieved by structural adjustment. During my experience as a physician I have never seen a negro suffer with chills and fever and have made extensive inquiry to ascertain whether the black race are subject to malaria. The answer has almost universally been "The colored man is immune." I have reasoned if this is so it is because the sun's rays are modified and fail to produce such effects when striking the negro's black skin, which in my mind is his protection.

SCARLET FEVER.

Definition of Scarlatina.—An acute contagious and exanthematous fever with a scarlet eruption, or rash; scarlet fever. It is probably caused by Class's bacillus, Diplococcus scarlatinae. It begins with chills, vomiting, and sore throat, followed by pyrexia and rapid pulse. After about twenty-four hours the eruption appears as a rash of thickly set red spots, which begin to fade in two or three days, and is often gone by the end of the first week. The fever departs in favorable cases with the disappearance of the eruption, which is attended by desquamation of the skin in fine branny scales and in large flakes. Recovery may often be looked for in two or three weeks, but is seldom complete in less than six weeks, and it is during this stage that kidney-complications are liable to occur, chiefly as a result of exposure to cold or wet. The nephritis is liable to lead to dropsy and uremia. Throat-, ear-, and eye-complications are not unfrequent, and often prove chronic. Scarlatina attacks principally children and youths, but may affect adults also. Second attacks are extremely rare.

—Dorland.

Symptoms and Etiology.—Scarlet fever is a disease as much or more dreaded by parents than are all other diseases of childhood because of the great mortality resulting therefrom. As a general thing all adults know what you mean when you speak of scarlet fever. Very few persons who have arrived at the age of man or womanhood can say they have never seen it. They all know how red the tongue, eyes, face and the skin of the upper part of the body appear during the first few days after it attacks the patient. All persons are familiar with the fact that there is much swelling of the glands of the throat, neck and the whole maxillary system. All know that often the inflammation of these glands is followed by pustular or gangrenous destruction and sloughing away of the parts with all the bad effects following such destruction.

It may be contagious but I think it more likely that it is the result of a poisonous gas which arises from the decomposition of fecal and other vegetable matter in places where drainage is imperfect (such as stables, privies

317

and pools of water that are close to the dwelling), and which is being inhaled by children who have had no chance to become infected by contact with other children who have the disease. During all my observation I have seen it attack and do its work with great fury in families whose children had no opportunity for such contact.

As the world knows all about the symptoms and its danger and as it is a matter of quarantine you should carry out all of the laws of the place in which you live governing this matter. It matters not to me as a mechanic whether this disease is contagious or epidemic. When I have a case to treat, the thing I want to know is what nerve, blood-vessel or gland has failed to perform its function and excrete poisonous products as fast as they accumulate? My object is to put the body in such condition that the glands of the excretory system of the entire body—the deep and superficial glands of the neck, those of the tongue, tonsils, fascia and skin, and also the kidneys—can carry off impurities before fermentation sets up. We must drive this poisonous fluid from the body as soon as possible or take the consequence, which is death.

When I am called to treat a case of scarlet fever I reason that the channels through which the arterial blood is delivered to the brain and those through which the venous blood is returned therefrom and which also drain the region of the tonsils, pharynx, larynx and the entire glandular system of the neck have become obstructed and the nerves in this region irritated, and muscular contractions have been set up. Thus we have blood retained in head, face and neck until partial or complete decomposition has gotten in its work and this is followed by the effects seen in the many symptoms known to belong to this disease.

Treatment.—I will now take up and give you what I consider the rational treatment of such diseases by a mechanic who knows the parts and principles of vital action as they exist in the human body. I know that I must remove all obstructions either by bones or contracted muscles that would in any way interfere with the delivery of arterial blood to the brain, and the entire glandular system of the head and neck, internal or external, the skin, the fascia, the lymphatics, the nerves, veins and arteries. They must each and all have their freedom if masterly work is expected from them.

Now I will begin my work at the atlas and proceed to the axis and all of the joints of the neck, the clavicles, the ribs and the vertebrae down to the

318

diaphragm. I generally sit on the side of the bed by the child as I do not wish to disturb him at all. I place my hand in the region of the lumbar because I want the kidneys, ureters and bladder to pass the waste products and all the fluids of this excretory system on and out without either obstruction or delay. We must adjust all articulations from the upper dorsal on down to and including the sacrum.

Make sure the splanchnic system is in full action because of its relation to the solar plexus. This is so important that we cannot afford to neglect it. Adjust the clavicles by bringing them fairly well forward in order to take all pressure or irritation off the arterial and nerve supply and the venous and lymphatic systems of drainage and renovation.

Now I place my hand under and back of the child's neck and gently pass my fingers round till they touch the transverse processes of the cervical vertebrae, then I place the fingers of the other hand behind the angle of the jaw and make a gentle easy separation of jaw and neck so that the blood can approach the brain, do its work and leave the brain with such impurities as it is expected to carry away. As to diet, in my opinion good nutritious soups for a few days are best for the patient. Plenty of fresh air and a good comfortable bed and bedding are all that is necessary. I use no salves, ointments or washes for the outside of the body or in the mouth and have seen no good results from outward or inward applications in scarlet fever. Follow this method, treating your patient at first from once to three times a day according to the severity of the case.

TYPHOID FEVER.

Definition.—Abdominal typhus, enteric fever, gastric fever; an acute febrile disease dependent upon entrance into the system of a specific microbe; it is attended by lesions of Peyer's patches, spleen, blood, and mesenteric glands, and accompanied by cerebral, abdominal, and thoracic symptoms. Toward the end of the first week rose-colored spots appear on the surface of the abdomen. It is not considered contagious in the ordinary sense, except so far as the excretions are concerned, the poison not being given off from the skin or in the breath, but in the faeces and urine.

—Dunglison.

Etiology and Examination.—We have nothing whatsoever that is absolute and trustworthy given us by the best medical writers concerning typhoid fever. They have failed to give us anything to guide us in cause hunting or to discover any trustworthy remedy or remedies. They speculate much about the typhoid bacillus, micro-organisms and so on but they overthrow that argument by saying the same bacilli are found in the healthy as well as in the unhealthy. So we give them credit for making a theory in one paragraph and then killing the same in the next. They administer all kinds of drugs, the mild and the most dangerous, such as mercury, strychnine, corrosive sublimate, alcohol and so on and finally say they have no hope for a successful combat with this deadly disease. They leave the impression that the medical doctor had as well stay at home and let the cook and the nurse have full charge of the typhoid cases.

This being the case the osteopath must be guided by the light of reason and ascertain in what part of the body a failure has appeared. As an engineer he must build his conclusions upon his knowledge of the cause and place of abnormal friction. If it is in the brain, heart, lungs, bowels or any organ, fascia, muscle or tissue or in the nervous system, say so, and when you speak show that you have obtained the truth by demonstration and do not lay the burden on to some imaginary bug or bacillus which is about as often found in the healthy as the unhealthy person.

The osteopath well knows that he must have two normally pure fluids, blood and nerve fluid. As a mechanical inspector he must travel through the entire digestive system on a hunt for such causes as would interfere with the production of pure arterial blood in quantities sufficient for all demands, or with the supply of nerve fluid to every organ. He should see that nothing interferes with the functioning of the blood and the nerve in the machinery of the body, through all of which they exercise and perform their functions separately and unitedly. Should he find a failure of the large intestine to prosecute to perfection the acts of reduction, separation to their original atomic condition and ab sorption of food products or to manufacture chyle and deliver it through the thoracic duct in sufficient quantity so that the lung can perfect pure arterial blood of the highest order for delivery through the heart to the abdominal viscera on time and in normal quantities—should we find this failure then what in your mind would be the natural question of the mechanic? Have the nerves to the colon failed to perform their function? If so seek the location and cause of that failure. If it is a partial dislocation of any bone or muscle that would result in pressure upon that part of the nervous system that supplies the colon then the operator can proceed and govern himself accordingly.

Allow me to draw your attention to the fact that in typhoid fever the conditions operating as causes are general and when I explore for them or such of the causes as would produce obstruction to any or all organs or the entire system, I begin at the occiput and search for any abnormal conditions of the bones and muscles of the neck because I know that such conditions produce irritation which would cause contracture of muscles and obstruction to blood and lymph vessels. Here I generally find heavy spasmodic contractures of the connecting muscles and ligaments which bear upon and confuse the nervous, arterial, venous and lymphatic systems resulting in a failure in their perfect circulation, a stagnation of fluids with an excess of impurities to be carried back for the lungs to renovate and repair and for the heart to return as arterial blood to keep in normal condition the cervical region and the head.

I reason that it is impossible to make good blood from bad or impure material. It is also impossible for the brain, when its own nourishment comes from a depleted arterial blood or is lessened by an inhibited drainage resulting in congestion, to supply normal healthy nerve fluid to the sympathetic ganglia so that they can carry out their functions. If we have diseased blood entering into the make-up of the arterial stream, when the stream should be pure, there will occur a shortage in functioning as a result.

In the upper dorsal of typhoid patients I generally find contracture of muscles strong enough to force the ribs so close together that the normal intercostal blood and nerve circulation is impossible. We must also consider the importance of the inferior cervical ganglion which when inhibited by pressure of rib, clavicle or muscle produces delay and stagnation in the nervous, venous and lymphatic currents.

We will now examine the ribs and vertebrae to and including the fifth, sixth, seventh and eighth dorsal. Here we find great rigidity of muscles, the ribs being drawn so closely together as to interfere with both blood and nerve supply to the intercostal muscles and to the spine also. From the region of the fifth and sixth we follow the great splanchnic nerves to the solar plexus to see what effect is produced, and we generally find the function of the semilunar ganglia disturbed. Also there is much soreness just below the sternum, back of and in the region of the stomach. As all the abdominal viscera without an exception are dependent upon the solar plexus for sensation, motion and nutrition, it is evident that here at the solar plexus is the place for us to halt in our spinal examination and trace out one by one the nerves that pass from the solar plexus to the stomach, pancreas, spleen, liver, kidneys, bladder, womb, omentum, peritoneum and bowels both great and small. If stagnation of fluid is followed by fermentation, inflammation and death both to the fluid and the part, have we not a mental lever that will raise the stomach and all tissues that cover the solar plexus and let you see at once that there is an irritation and constriction from the center of the solar plexus to the termination of all branches leaving the center to execute functional action in the whole abdomen, nothing excepted?

With this fact before us can we expect anything but imperfect digestion and the collection of imperfect fluid to be carried to the heart and lungs to make future blood? With reason we will arrive at the conclusion that no good blood can be produced from the poisonous compounds generated in the organs of the abdomen and thrown together into the receptaculum chyli and conducted by way of the heart to the lungs. Would we as mechanics show our ignorance of this fact while in the sick room of the suffering patient or would we proceed to gently lift or raise the stomach, omentum and all tis sues up-

and off of the solar plexus, the aorta, the vena cava and the whole nerve and blood system of the abdomen, and not waste time hunting for typhoid germs? Give freedom to the solar plexus and it will soon furnish a germicide that will drive the bugaboos from the system by the way of the lungs, the kidneys, the skin and the bowels.

Continuing we will explore the region of the ninth, tenth, eleventh and twelfth ribs which we generally find in a relaxed condition and lying far back and producing pressure on the nerves and blood-vessels which supply the entire renal system, the kidneys, the ureters and the bladder. Thus far my examination has been directed chiefly to the patient's right side. Now let us give special attention to the left side, beginning at the neck. Examine carefully all bones till the clavicle is reached which we often find far in toward the neck or too far back on the acromian process. We also find some of the upper ribs varied from their normal positions by contractions of muscles that extend from neck to the spine and ribs. Now we will proceed to make sure that the fifth, sixth, seventh and eighth vertebrae and ribs are not interfering with the blood and nerve supply which passes between them, and that there is no muscular contracture which brings the ribs too close together. I make a special exploration of the left side because I want normal action of heart and spleen, as well as kidney and ureter of this side.

I am very careful on this side in dealing with typhoid patients to know that all is correct. From the ninth rib on down to the lumbar I explore very carefully, for the reason that many causes might operate here that would irritate the quadratus lumborum and other muscles that attach to these ribs and would pull the ribs from their normal positions. I reason that normality of position is necessary to good health and any abnormal position of bone or muscle would produce the opposite condition.

Treatment.—When I am called to a case and enter the room to find a typhoid fever patient I realize at once that I have universal stagnation to deal with. I know this stagnation is the effect of inhibition of nerve and blood circulation. I begin my treatment by adjusting the atlas and all of the bones of the neck to the truly normal. When there is much muscular rigidity I inhibit the nerves in the region, both front and back of the neck. After this is done I adjust the clavicles to their normal articulations at both ends. I see that the hyoid bone is free from muscle contractures. I adjust the scapula by raising it up so that the serratus magnus and all the ribs to which it is attached are normal in position. I spread the arms apart after which I bring the arms one at a time close to the side and taking hold at the elbow push them up in order to free up the axillary system.

When I find any of the upper ribs too far back, which is usually the case as is shown by the bulging, I bring or pull those ribs forward simply by placing one hand under the scapula holding the ribs firmly and then bring the arm out at right angles—well out and down, gently but firmly, to loosen up all the muscles attached to the scapula and free up both nerve and blood circulation. Now I proceed to adjust the fifth, sixth, seventh and eighth when they are found out of line. Then I go on to the ninth, tenth, eleventh and twelfth adjusting any abnormal bone, muscle or ligament.

In the lumbar region I usually find the fourth and fifth vertebrae too far back. Sometimes the entire lumbar is abnormally convex which I adjust as the patient lies on the bed by placing my hands underneath the back, fingers on the transverse processes and pull them up so as to reduce any posterior luxation affecting the kidneys or bladder. Treat your patient daily. Be governed by the severity of the case. When you are called in early treat from one to three times a day, then as symptoms subside I treat once or twice a day as the needs of the case demand. As recovery is apparent or assured diminish the number of treatments.

In very severe cases I have made it a rule to fill the bowels with a gruel made from flour well heated till it turns a light yellow, then make a quart of gruel and add one half pint of cream (not milk). I inject one half of this quantity into the lower bowel then in six hours inject the remainder. I do this because I find that the whole nutrient system is laboring under starvation.

TYPHUS FEVER.

Definition.—Putrid, jail, hospital, or ship fever, petechial, maculated, or spotted fever. Acute febrile disease dependent upon the entrance into the system of a specific microbe; characterized by high temperature, small, weak, but usually frequent pulse, with great prostration of strength and much cerebral disturbance; its duration is usually a fortnight to three weeks or longer. It is marked by lesions of the blood, but not of organs; is endemic, epidemic, and highly contagious.

—*Dunglison.*

Etiology.—I have given you Dunglison's definition of what is generally known to be typhus, or jail fever, and I would suggest that the osteopath add to this definition, filth fever. While we will not disagree with the medical authors on the contagious nature of typhus, we will go a little farther and say that when sanitation is observed and its laws carried out by thoroughly cleaning up all dirt and filth, this disease prevails very little if at all. This filth accumulates, ferments, decomposes and throws off poisonous gases, and it is easy enough to reason that the person who eats, drinks and sleeps in the vicinity of such filth-produced gas or gases will have some kind of abnormal disturbance due to such inhalations. This fact is too well known by every one for me to take up your time detailing laboratory stories of the peculiar micro-organisms, bacteria and so on, that are said to be found in the blood, the sputum, the urine and the fecal matter of typhus fever patients.

Since 1861 I have known for a certainty that human beings cannot breathe the gases that are thrown off from decaying animals without going through the process of dysentery followed by a fever which is the effort of Nature to deliver the body from poisonous substances generated by inhaling such gases. This I well know because in 1861 when in the army the regiment I was in camped in a field where fifteen or twenty horses had been killed some five or six days previously in the hot September weather. Now while there was not the least perceptible breeze in motion I could feel waves of this invisible subtile gas pass over my face and I drew the attention of the doctors to the fact asking if they could feel this wave passing over their faces while they were lying on the ground during the night. They said they not only felt the wave but noticed a peculiar sweetish odor which came from those horses. These horses were bloated as tight as the hides could hold. About three days later fully one third of the regiment fell sick with dysentery followed by fever. I knew nothing of osteopathy then and did not think for an instant that the inhaling of such decomposing animal gases could produce a shock which would reach to the storehouse or headquarters of the nerve fluid, constrict and interfere with not only the pneumogastric nerve but the whole nervous system as well as the blood and other fluids of the entire body. Since then the mystery of the why of such fevers as typhus and scarlet fever and enteric disturbances has been cleared up by the fact that in such sickness I have always found some such decomposing substances either in the house, yard, well or some place close by the sleeping apartments of those who have fallen ill.

I pay no attention to laboratory stories of microorganisms. I have no time to spend or to reason about what Professors A and B have seen under their microscopes in specimens taken from the body of a man, after death and decomposition have done their work. The instruments that I use in my laboratory when seeking for the cause and relief of typhus fever are spades, pitchforks, water and fire to dispose of all filth. It takes no microscope to see a dead cat, a dead dog, a lot of old boots and shoes, dishes holding stagnant water, unclean chamber utensils, kitchen filth around the back door, and so on. Be sure you take your spade and pitchfork into the cellar, yard and out-houses, turn and rest not until you can say, after having put your nose to the ground and smelt, that you have found the filth producing the poison. After you have seen to a thorough cleaning up of the house, out-buildings, yards and surroundings, enter the house and see that all bedding, clothing and so on are taken out into the fresh air and sunshine. Then burn some wool or burn some sugar and fill the house with the smoke therefrom. Start a little fire in the stove or fire place in order to secure an active draft and draw your imaginary microbes up the chimney. Now you have your sanitary condition secured and the filth abolished. You are ready to give your patient osteopathic treatment which will be of no account to him unless he is worked upon by a mechanic.

The gases operating as poisons must be totally destroyed, as the inhalation of such gases stagnates the whole nervous system. The osteopath must know that the nervous system of a patient who has inhaled such gases for days, weeks, and in some cases for months, is overcome by being loaded down with poisonous fluids to such a degree that the entire excretory system has become powerless to carry on the necessary healthy renovation. When searching for causes remember to examine wells and cisterns. Often a cat, dog or hen gets into a well and is not discovered until sickness and death result.

Treatment.—My method of treatment in typhus fever has no mysteries about it. It has been successful for thirty-five years, hence satisfactory to me and also to my patient. I care nothing at all for analysis of urine or sputum. Neither do I care for the temperature or the pulse whether they are high or low. My object has always been to begin with the nervous system which is supplied from the brain. I know that before the brain can manufacture the necessary fluids it must not only have plenty of good arterial blood but also no stagnant venous blood. Hence my first effort is to open the doors through which arterial blood should pass to the brain.

I examine and adjust the union of the neck with the head, and the articulation of the inferior maxillary bone just the same as I do in measles, mumps and other glandular diseases. If I do my duty the arterial blood will reach the brain and there will be no obstruction by contracted muscles or any variation of atlas, axis or other bones of the neck. Then when I know I have the arterial channels open I am just as careful to know that the venous system has free and unobstructed drainage. Success is always shown by the fulness of the jugular veins. They begin to fill as soon as normal blood action is established to and from the brain. I continue the exploration and adjustment all along the neck and the entire extent of the spine to the sacrum and coccyx.

By this time the student may think that I put in a great deal of time talking about the atlas, the axis, the spine, ribs, clavicles and the scapulae in most of these diseases. It matters but little to me what is thought or said; give me a patient with a good heart, a good brain, with an open road between and I will give you a healthy person in a few days instead of the sick one who is laboring under some of these so-called mysterious diseases, in which the anatomical engineer fails to find any mystery but does find the result of stagnation of the fluids of the body, the effect of inhaling poisonous gases. In the condition called typhus fever my object is to get both the nerve and blood systems free from any constriction in order that the processes of renovation and repair can go on, resulting in complete health. As to beds, use such as the patient has been accustomed to and is comfortable in, and good clean sheets and covers. Have plenty of good fresh air in the room. Give such nutritious easily digested food as is ordinarily used and this is all I have to say on diet.

What I have given you in reference to treatment is intended to apply to patients to whom you have been called in the early stages of the disease when the patient has been sick but a few-days. If I am called in to treat cases that have had the fever for a number of weeks and I find much prostration I adjust the best I can all bones from the head to the coccyx. When there is great exhaustion, tremulous condition and wandering of mind I proceed to fill the colon, which I consider is in a starved condition, with a nutritious gruel made from flour (not starch) which is first exposed in a skillet to just enough heat to overcome the tendency to ferment and to turn it a light yellow. Make of it one quart of gruel and add one half a pint of sweet cream. Inject about one pint of this gruel into the lower bowel and in from four to six hours inject the remainder. This treatment I follow up by a similar injection every other day should it be necessary. I find this sufficient to re-establish nutrition in the colon.

BILIOUS FEVER.

Definition.—One with apparent liver-complications and attended with the vomiting of bile.   —*Dorland*.

Symptoms.—Bilious fever is too well known and understood by those living in the Western and Middle States and particularly so by the pioneers to require a lengthy description of how it appears and proceeds to get in its work. It generally appears during the latter part of August or September and between 36 and 46 degrees north latitude. It is usually preceded for a few days by a tired, weak feeling of the whole system. The limbs feel weak. There is a weighty feeling of the stomach and abdomen, sometimes a running off at the bowels for a few days. This is followed by a chill, headache, backache, particularly in the lumbar region. After this chill passes off fever follows with vomiting of a great deal of bilious matter. There is high colored urine, dry and heavily coated tongue. You can call this bilious fever, or fall fever.

Etiology.—The operator knows when he has bilious fever to contend with from the bilious matter thrown off and the high colored urine. He knows that the excretory system has been interfered with and has come to a halt. The system is performing the chemical action necessary in producing bilious matter, and its retention is the cause of this poisonous irritation of the system and he must help his patients get rid of it if he wishes to relieve and cure them. The medical doctor would puke, purge, sweat his patient and give him quinine and opiates in order to remove the bilious matter from the system. The osteopathic mechanic would commence his search for obstructing causes at the lumbar region. Here he finds variations from a truly normal condition. He reasons that the spinal muscles have been relaxed by the powerful heat of the sun. He finds the lumbar bulging backwards. He goes further up and finds the lower ribs prolapsed and pressing on the renal nerves. He goes higher up and finds the great splanchnic nerves squeezed and pressed upon by the ribs which have become relaxed and dropped down from their articulations with the fifth, sixth, seventh and eighth dorsal vertebrae. He passes on up to the first, second, third and fourth or upper dorsals. He finds them like the lumbar, too far back producing another hump.

Treatment.—If your patient is an adult place him in the knee-chest position using a narrow, long stool which is about twelve inches high under the chest and give him a thorough spinal treatment from coccyx to the dorsal region as has been described many times in this book. Then adjust every variation from the normal clear up to the occiput. Follow this treatment from once to three times a day until all fever and misery have left the body and normal action of the kidneys, bowels, stomach and nervous system has been secured. After this treatment, once or twice a week or in ten days is sufficient. Let your patient have a good plain wholesome diet. See that he keeps out of the sun especially from its hot rays between ten and four o'clock.

When there is much headache I am very particular to adjust the atlas, axis and on through the cervical vertebrae down to the fifth dorsal, which universally gives relief if properly done. I am sure to keep all drugs out of the system. When you follow this method I think you will be satisfied with the results. I have had no trouble in handling bilious fever.

YELLOW FEVER.

Definition.—An acute infectious disease of warm latitudes characterized by tenderness in the epigastrium, jaundice, constipation, vomiting (often of altered blood, "black vomit"), fever, and albuminuria; the dis ease is undoubtedly caused by the presence of a microorganism, probably protozoan, but this has not yet been isolated; it is communicated from the sick to the well by the agency of a mosquito.

—Dunglison.

General Discussion.—I do not expect to dwell on the cause producing such conditions as are called by the name of yellow fever because I have never lived in the latitudes or localities in which yellow fever prevails. I am satisfied that it prevails between the Equator and 26 degrees north latitude. From 26 to 36 degrees what is known as bilious fever seems to take the place of yellow fever as to latitude. From 36 to 46 degrees I have observed a mixture of bilious fever, flux and chills and fever. From 46 to 56 degrees we have more of the typhoid, mountain fever, pneumonia and tuberculosis.

My attention was called to the effect of latitude as an etiologic factor in such diseases as this by a government surveyor in 1843 or '44. As I remember it his name was Captain Brent. At that time he was surveying north Missouri running the range for township lines. He was doing this work in the hot weather during the latter part of the summer. He was a man about six feet tall and had a very fair skin. He spoke of the yellow fever, bilious fever, chills and fever, mountain fever and so on. He said that such fevers were con fined to latitudes as I have given you or at least very much so. He thought from his observation that the latitude and the direct or modified rays of the sun had much to do in producing these conditions. This was of much interest to me as I had never seen or treated yellow fever but had many years' experience with bilious fever, chills and fever and such diseases as prevail between 36 and 46 degrees north latitude. I was well acquainted with the symptoms and the treatment medically, before the birth of osteopathy which was in 1874, after which date I began to reason and experiment with these conditions and also with flux and cholera morbus along the lines of mechanics or osteopathy. To my surprise at that time I found that such fevers could be successfully treated

331

by mechanical adjustment of the spine and ribs from the sacrum to the occiput. I found that fever, dysentery, headache and all this kind of suffering were ready to yield to osteopathic treatment. After opening my school I spoke freely of this to my classes in order to prove and demonstrate that even though there was little to hope for in the use of medicine in such diseases that there was not only hope but relief and cure by the simple process of normalizing the framework of the human body. I have since seen quite a number of the graduates of my school who have been in Cuba, the Philippines and other places where yellow fever prevails. They have all reported good success as the result of osteopathic treatment for all those tropical fevers. One of my lady graduates while in the Philippines with her son who was an officer in the army gave, as she afterward told me, many treatments to the soldiers, notwithstanding neither she nor the soldiers treated felt called upon to say anything to the doctors about it and that the results were always satisfactory. Other osteopaths report successful work done in Cuba. For further particulars in regard to treatment see bilious fever. I advise all my graduates to observe carefully all laws governing quarantine and in treating your patient adjust the body the entire length of the spine and so take the fever down.

RELAPSE.

Definition.—(Relabor, to fall back). The return of a disease during or shortly after convalescence.

—*Dunglison.*

Many persons after having to all appearances recovered from an attack of typhus, bilious fever, over heat, flux, dysentery, chills and fever, or other disease producing great nervous prostration, have a return of the condition due to over exertion, exposure, fatigue or over-loading the stomach while the system is weak from the preceding attack. I call this condition relapsing fever. When you are called to treat a case of relapse, I will say for the benefit of the operator that you have a case of fluid stagnation of the whole system. The nerve supply is exhausted and the blood supply impure and oppressive to the whole nervous system because it has been retained long enough to be in a state of fermentation.

Treatment.—I begin with the patient's spine and treat it just as I did to relieve him of the original fever. I carefully adjust the articulations of the neck, the dorsal, the lumbar and ribs. Also I am very particular while my patient is lying on his back to set at liberty the arterial and venous circulation in the region of the solar plexus for I know that the whole abdomen is weak and exhausted. I am careful when a patient is in the knee chest position to bring up from the pelvis the lower bowels and other organs as far up as the kidneys. I do this in order that the excretory system may begin and do the important work of liberating the body from all elements that should be conducted from it by way of the kidneys. With what I have given in reference to treatment in typhoid cases as a guide I think I have said enough about this condition.

UNCLASSIFIED.

MISCELLANEOUS SUBJECTS.

ENLARGED PROSTATE GLAND.

I have found the ischia too close together in all cases of enlarged prostate glands that I have examined and treated in the past thirty years. In all these cases I have given relief and brought about a reduction of the enlarged gland by the simple process of spreading the ischia apart. If such cases have gone on to ulceration or cancerous sloughing, then the osteopath may be justified in the use of his knife. As a rule good results follow when the ischia are brought back and kept in their normal positions at their articulations with the sacrum.

BOILS AND CARBUNCLES.

Definition of Furunculus.—Boil; furuncle. Small phlegmon appearing under the form of a conical hard, circumscribed tumor, having its seat in the dermal texture. After an uncertain period it becomes pointed, white or yellow, and gives exit to pus mixed with blood. When it breaks, a small, grayish, fibrous mass some times appears, consisting of dead areolar tissue; this is called the core, ventriculus, or nucleus furunculi. The abscess does not heal until after its separation. The indications of treatment are to discuss by the application of leeches and warm fomentations, or to encourage suppuration by warm, emollient cataplasms. When suppuration is entirely established the part may be opened or suffered to break, according to circumstances. A blind boil is an indolent, imperfectly suppurating, phlegmonous tumor, of the kind described above, often seated in a sebaceous follicle, as in acne indurata.

—Dunglison.

Definition of Carbuncle.—1. An inflammation of the subcutaneous tissue, terminating in a slough and in suppuration, and accompanied by marked constitutional symptoms. The swelling is at first covered by a tight,

335

reddened skin, which later becomes thin and perforated by a number of openings discharging pus. This mass finally sloughs away, leaving an ulcerated excavation. 2. A whelk or lump on the face.

—*Dorland.*

Some of those pus-forming tumors in the skin such as boils are the result of stagnant venous blood ac cumulating from lack of circulation. Nature's process of freeing the skin from this blood is a chemical action called fermentation which produces pus. Boils appear on any part of the body and if not irritated by bruising will naturally come to a head and make an outlet for the pus. The less interference there is the sooner it will ripen and burst. In a few days there generally comes out a plug or core which is the dead skin. When a boil should be opened thrust the point of a lance through the yellow part. Evacuation of its contents will follow. After the boil has discharged its contents ointments are generally applied, but I think it is better to use a wet cloth, because of the hydrogen and oxygen in the water.

Sometimes boils or abscesses extend to the fascia of the neck, face or any part of the body. It is better to keep the lance out of boils of this kind as long as possible particularly those of the neck. Sometimes they appear on or in the fingers and are called felons. When I am satisfied pus is formed I slip a lance through the side of the finger and beneath the tendon or muscle, but never through the tendon. The knife can be passed close to the bone to let out the pus and dead blood without disfiguring the fingers. Boils or abscesses on the fingers come from blows or bruises and the sooner the blood is let out the better, for it prevents protracted inflammation and sloughing off of the muscles and tendons. If there is dead blood lying between the bone and tendon of the affected finger, keep a moist cloth over the wound for a day or two after drainage is established in order to keep up drainage.

I would advise you to be very careful of carbuncles in the neck particularly if they are very deep seated. Place your patient on the side and keep wet cloths on the neck until matter forms and comes to a head. Be patient until the skin gets thin enough for you to make a small incision for the evacuation of the pus. Such carbuncles are better off without the use of the knife. Generally several openings are formed out of which pus will ooze. Wet cloths applied are better than salves or poultices because the skin is swelled so tight it absorbs nothing. Following the application of the wet cloths oily plasters such as are generally used will do as a dressing until the healing process is completed.

TETANUS.

Definition.—Spasm with rigidity. A disease consisting in a permanent contraction of all the muscles, or merely of some, without alternations of relaxation, characterized by closure of the jaws, difficulty or impracticability of deglutition, rigidity and immobility of the limbs and trunk, which is sometimes curved forward (emprosthotonos), sometimes backward (opisthotonos), sometimes to one side (pleurothotonos). When confined to the muscles of the jaws it is called trismus. Traumatic tetanus is that which supervenes on a wound. When occurring in the puerperal condition it is called puerperal tetanus, tetanus puerperarum. A tetanic contraction of single muscles does not imply necessarily the general disease or the action of the specific cause. A specific anaerobic microorganism is credited with the production of the disease.

—Dunglison.

In all punctures of hand, foot, or body at any point or place, made by toy pistols or any other object, if I have any fear of tetanus from the wound the first thing I do is to wash the wound and the part for some distance around it. Then wring a towel or other cloth out of water and wrap it around the wounded part for some distance and pour plenty of alcohol on the wet bandage. I keep this on the wound for a few hours then I dilute the alcohol with water, about one half water, and continue to apply this for a few hours or days. The misery of the wound generally begins to disappear inside of one hour. Follow this up for twenty-four hours or longer if the misery should re appear. This has been my method for many years and I have never lost a case that I treated after this method. My object was to prevent lockjaw and so far I have had uniform success. I have had nail or other punctures of the hand and foot yield to this treatment after the inflammation had almost reached the elbow or knee. In these cases the bandage should cover the arm to the elbow and the leg to the knee. The fever, pain and misery would leave the limb and the patient would turn over and go to sleep.

I think the spasmodic contracture in these cases is from magnetic action of the muscles and my object is to overcome the power of this magnetic force that is holding the muscles together, and so far the wet towel and alcohol has given relief.

HYDROPHOBIA.

Definition.—Rabies; an infectious disease communicated by the bites of animals affected with rabies, and believed to be due to a micro-organism which is as yet undiscovered. After an incubation-period of from one to six months the disease begins with malaise, depression of spirits, and swelling of the lymphatics in the region of the wound. There is choking and spasmodic catching of the breath, succeeded by increasing tetanio spasms, especially of the muscles of respiration and deglutition, which is increased by attempts to drink water or even by the sight of water. There are usually also fever, mental derangement, vomiting, profuse secretion of a sticky saliva, and albuminuria. The disease is generally fatal, death occurring in from two to five days.

—Dorland.

I believe the dog shows much lime in his fecal and urinary discharges, and what we call hydrophobia is the result of a peculiar lime poison that comes from the dog. To prevent it my object is to first neutralize the poisonous saliva of the dog. To do this I make a solution of sulphuric acid, about twenty parts water and one of the acid. I wash the wound in this solution, and if severe, I apply wet cloths saturated in the solution.

Many years ago while I was in Kansas there was a mad dog which passed through the neighborhood and bit a colt, a calf, some hogs and a young lady. With his teeth he tore two gashes in her face from the cheek bone down to the under jaw. For ten days I gave her the treatment above indicated. She is alive and well yet. The animals bitten died with hydrophobia.

I gave the same treatment to a young man who was bitten on the foot by a supposed hydrophobic dog. He lived several years afterwards and showed no signs of hydrophobia. Take this suggestion for treatment for what it is worth.

SNAKE BITE.

The bite of a rattle snake has a very different effect from that of a mad dog, producing much watery swelling which I think is the effect of an acid virus. I have always treated the snake bite with alkalies, I prefer spirits of ammonia. I open the wound freely and fill it at once with the ammonia. When I cannot get the ammonia I take good soda. Wet it so as to make a poultice and cover the wound with it. I take my knife and work the soda into the bottom of the wound. I have treated many cases and the progress of the swelling stopped in a very short time, not over an hour in any case. I give my experience as I think it may be of some benefit to the reader.

OSTEOPATHY AND THE SOLIDITY OF ITS FOUNDATION.

As the discoverer of the Science of Osteopathy I named the school which I founded at Kirksville, Mo., the American School of Osteopathy because from start to finish it is distinctly an American product. It is a product of North America and particularly of the United States where the people think, reason and act upon their own judgment. There are wise and able thinkers all over the United States. I think their pioneer life has had much to do in qualifying them to reason from cause to effect and from effect to cause especially along the line of inventions. They use the English language to convey their ideas and with it can well be described any science or discovery made by man from his advent to the present day.

My ancestors had in their veins the blood of the English, the Scotch and the German, but I think we have just as able men and women in North America as in Europe. The English speaking race has everywhere shown superiority in inventive genius and the power of thought. In this country, freedom of thought, speech and action has been without restraint since the words "All men are free and equal" were written. Liberty of speech is man's God-given right. We think, reason, conclude and act upon that conclusion without asking whether it pleases the rulers or the people. We are bold to show the work and let it stand on its own merit. We feel that if Europe wants to appropriate any of our products either physical or mental they have a right to do so. We are willing to hear their approval or disapproval, also their prophesies on the durability of the science or work.

In 1874 was raised the banner of Osteopathy on which was written a demonstrable science which is taking the place of the systems of the healing art which are unreliable in diagnosis, prognosis and treatment of diseases of all kinds. In thirty-five years it has grown from infancy to manhood never having met with a single obstruction or reverse, notwithstanding would-be prophets said it would soon die and its place be known no more forever. Such prophesies have even found a place in osteopathic journals but the speed of the progress of osteopathy has increased every year, day and hour since June 22, 1874. As an American I am proud to know that every day the sun rises, it shines upon more brilliant osteopathic thinkers and upon more persons who have thrown away their crutches and pills. I am glad that the osteopaths from all schools can show by their work that their philosophy is true. They have met with much opposition because of the merited success of their work. With the M. D. it is not a question of whether osteopathy is true or false, but whether his patients will leave him and go to the mechanical engineer who knows what part of the human body is ab normal and producing the affliction. The ability of osteopathy to give relief and cure has been sufficiently demonstrated in cases where medicine has acknowledged its inability to produce the desired result—health.

I suppose by a rough guess there are over worthy osteopaths in the field who have a good practice and are being well paid for their services. Your good work is the soul and body of your success both in restoring your patient to health and in getting plenty of money for your services. From my experience I think that he who depends upon the patients he has cured for his advertising is far better off than the man who depends upon the traveling osteopathic lecturer who tells what wonderful men the "Old Doctor" and his boys are. Go to work, tend to your business and you will find that if you cure an asthmatic, a case of goiter, shaking palsy, lameness of spine or limbs, those grateful patients will do more advertising for you than a dozen traveling lecturers. My advice is to let your object be to keep out of papers and do good work today and better work tomorrow and your patients will multiply just in proportion to your ability to demonstrate that you know your business.

For thirty-five years I have kept my name out of papers as much as possible. I have been visited and solicited by reporters hundreds of times to let them give me a write up which would cost me the small sum of fifty or one hundred dollars according to the size of the paper. I have told all such to keep my name out of papers and let my work stand for itself.

LIFE.

One of the greatest questions, if not the greatest, that has ever presented itself to any philosopher in any age is, what is life? Is life a substance? If so what are its attributes? He reasons on the attributes of known substances such as electricity. What are its attributes if any? Electricity shows its attributes to be force and motion. Is there any substance whose attributes are superior to electricity? At the end of all his philosophical labors the philosopher concludes that life is a substance and superior to the sum total of the elements of the whole universe. Its superiority is proven by one of its attributes which is mind. Mind by its unlimited skill rules, governs and uses at will all forces and elements. The ability of mind is shown by its power to rule and govern all forces wisely and to prepare, construct and manage the motion of this and all other worlds of the universe. By the attribute of mental action, life plans, specifies, prepares, constructs the world and its inhabitants, vegetable, mineral and animal and brings them under the control of all elements of motion necessary for their preparation and construction.

Thus the philosopher reasons that the universe is governed by the attributes of the substance known as life. We say "The living God," and what are His attributes but the sum total of all knowledge to rule and govern all parts and principles that are governed by any law of intelligence. Thus he concludes that life is a substance that as a substance has attained the degree of perfection, and that life and intelligence are universal and unlimited in extent, time and power. If this is not his conclusion he does not give life and its attributes the credit their work merits.

Let us mention a few of the forces of Nature life, electricity, oxygen and air. These are all individual substances. As life is as plentiful as oxygen, filling all space and each and every atom of the universe, we will work to keep conditions in line and wait results. One says that the atom enters the germ cell. How does it receive life while in that cell? As life is as universal as electricity and will act equally as quick when the battery is in working order then we will look for life to appear in all substances when the proper connection is made. Life is there and will show its presence when brought in contact with the battery. Life is a sub stance which fills all of the space of the whole universe.

One of its attributes is action under all proper conditions. It gives form and motion to both physical and intellectual. One of its powers is to select the kind of matter that will make flesh to suit any fiber or muscle in man, beast, bird, reptile, or that will make mineral, vegetable, all gases, fluids, and the forces of all Nature. It selects and adjusts and supplies life to atoms, beings, worlds and keeps them equipped with material and motion, with mind to construct and wisdom to govern all motions of the body formed by its eternal labors. Life is the God, the wisdom, the power and the motion of all.

As oxygen is a well-known substance with qualities peculiar to itself and which fills the place in Nature that all vitality depends on and without which animal and vegetable could not exist, we are led to look for life and see if it is not an individualized substance also and learn if it has qualities and powers superior to oxygen, electricity and other substances over which it seems to have universal power and control in the economy of Nature. If we find such to be true then we can work with better results as healers. The bone, muscle, nerve, blood, hair and all fluids of the body are visible facts. On general principles we know their forms, places and uses, but as to how or by what process the blood passed from food to flesh we are at sea and will be so until we find the process the arterial blood passes through to prepare the atom to unite with life and take its place and obey the demand of mind and motion.

LIFE IS DUAL.

In the union of any two elements we have a cause producing an effect, a new being superior to either element in the compound. Unite hydrogen with oxygen, the result is water, a new being. We find in man and beast that previous to the formation of a new being there must be a union of two lives. We know that the life of one being is not sufficient to form another being. Thus we are prepared to see that one of the attributes of life is that the union of living forces is demanded for the formation of a body. In the union of the male and female elements we have a child. Unite the male life substance with the higher life substance of the female and the effect is known by the product. I think life in all animals is dual because of the difference there is in the parents. In the male, the compound is different from that of the female and by the union of their lives, though different in attributes, we have a case resulting in taking from general life and producing a new being of any animal species. Thus in all animals we have an organized being, a new product, the result of the union of living forces. From this union we get mind as the ruling attribute.

LIFE IN FORM.

When we address a person by speech we expect an answer from his power of reason, expressed by action of his vocal organs. We know he speaks, but by what process did his organs make the sound and form the words of the answer? Has his life a form? If so we can expect it to act accordingly. Then we will hunt for its attributes. If we find mind is one of them then the mystery vanishes. For to me reason, which we expect to answer us, is an effect whose cause is mental action and the reply is the demonstration, or life using its attributes to think, conclude, and report to you by its vocal machinery which is made to suit the production of varied sounds. Talk would fail to be heard and understood if the organized being of life were not at the helm. I can think of life in each person as the being who makes the body of man and places all organs under its system of perfect action, both mental and physical. Life in man is itself a man and the body is the empire he controls. The region of the heart is his headquarters where all orders effecting the whole living government, man's body, are given and received.

CONCLUSION.

If the body is the empire of the living man how large is the emperor? Is it necessary for him to be as large as the whole empire? Is not the house much larger than the lady who presides over and governs it? As we know that is true we will have to reason that life in man and beast is an organized being of per feet purity of material and mind with powers so great that but little space in the body is required. My opinion is that organized life in man or beast is very small and is the power behind the throne of man's physical body.

A FINAL EXHORTATION.

The machinist or engineer who would conduct the human body from the abnormal condition which is disease, to the normal which is health and happiness, must think and do as a mechanic or his effort will be a failure. The theoretical blank has no place in this day of independent thought. He who runs a bicycle, an automobile or any machine designed for locomotion or other purposes must acquaint himself with the parts, and the whole machine, before he can run it with safety to himself and others. This is the day when man's useful education is the practical. The time has come for the practical man to lay down all undemonstrable theories and prove what he says by what he does. He cannot afford to be a laughing stock for those who know and are governed by the absolute laws of Nature, the laws that have been demonstrated in steam, electricity and all professions by such men as will not walk in the footsteps of past days in the pursuit of any subject sacred or profane. The original thinker on any subject cares nothing for so-called authority either of the past or present. He does not care for the priest, pope, president, czar, emperor, sultan or any authority but one and that is the God of Nature who proves His perfection by His architecture, His plan, His specification, His building and engineering of all the mechanism of the solar and planetary systems and all of their works. That Philosopher, that Mechanic and Engineer is the only Author to whom I pay homage. Keep your mud valves open and your engine in such condition that you can move out of the hearing of theories, and halt for all coming days by the side of the river of the pure waters of reason and be able to demonstrate that which you assert. The more we know of the architecture of the God of Nature, and the closer we follow it the better we will be pleased with the results of our work.